"Drawing on a wealth of cultural and clinical experience, Koichi Togashi's innovative new book is a welcome and necessary addition to contemporary psychoanalysis, a field that is shaped by its Western outlook. The decolonizing impulse at the heart of *The Psychoanalytic Zero* is a refreshing and vital contribution. Togashi introduces us to different ways of thinking, thereby challenging our traditional assumptions and enriching our knowledge about human experience and analytic practice."

—**Roger Frie**, Ph.D., Psy.D., Professor at Simon Fraser University and Psychoanalytic Faculty and Supervisor, William Alanson White Institute, New York

"A thoughtful and challenging voice from Japan, Koichi Togashi provides a fundamental alternative to the Western presumptions of traditional psychoanalysis. Illustrating his perspective with wonderful clinical storytelling, he invites us to 'decolonize' psychoanalysis and open ourselves to the challenges of emptiness. This book is for therapists and students ready to ask big questions, and keeps us absorbed. A true gift from the East."

—**Donna M. Orange**, New York University Postdoctoral Program in Psychoanalysis and Psychotherapy, author, *Psychoanalysis, History, and Radical Ethics: Learning to Hear*

"By refocusing our vision eastward toward Asia, Koichi Togashi brings a fresh and thoroughly innovative perspective to many aspects of the psychoanalytic situation. Starting with the premise that 'being precedes awareness' he shows how 'the psychoanalytic zero' which has its roots in the Heart Sutra of Mayahana Buddhism as well as *Taoism*, decenters psychoanalysis from the iron grip of Western thought and values. Togashi confronts the reader with the startling awareness that such familiar topics as trauma, guilt, and responsibility take on new meaning when viewed through an Eastern lens. But perhaps even more importantly, reading this book allows the reader to find new answers to questions about what it means to be human."

—**Doris Brothers**, co-founder of The Training and Research in Intersubjective Self Psychology Foundation, advisory board and council of the IAPSP

THE PSYCHOANALYTIC ZERO

The Psychoanalytic Zero: A Decolonizing Study of Therapeutic Dialogues is written from the unique perspective of a Western-trained Asian psychoanalyst and applies principles of Eastern philosophy to understand the psychoanalytic relationship, psychoanalytic processes, and their uses—and limitations—for alleviating human suffering.

Bringing a unique Eastern perspective to a previously Western-dominated discipline and framed within the current relational and ethical trends in psychoanalysis, the book enables readers to develop a language for understanding an Eastern ethical viewpoint and explore how this language can change our awareness of psychoanalytic practice and human suffering. Chapters are devoted to the Eastern concepts of nothingness, emptiness, surrender, sincerity, silence and narrative, and issues including existential "guilt of being," trauma, contingency, informed consent, the sense of being human, and uncertainty. Discussions are illustrated and illuminated through vivid recreations and careful elaboration of therapeutic case studies with traumatized patients. The studies demonstrate the process by which patients regain a sense of being human. This enriched perspective will, it is hoped, help the analyst treat traumatized patients who are unable to relate to others, and who do not experience themselves as being human.

The Psychoanalytic Zero will enrich an analyst's sensitivity to the appearance of the moment without context—the psychoanalytic zero—which opens infinite opportunities for continued growth in a psychoanalytic relationship. It will be of great appeal to psychoanalysts and psychoanalytic psychotherapists interested in self-psychological, intersubjective, and relational theories.

Koichi Togashi, Ph.D., L.P., is a Professor at Konan University, Kobe, Japan, and a Faculty and Training and Supervising Analyst at TRISP, New York, U.S.A. He works in private practice in Kobe and Hiroshima, Japan.

Like its counterpart, *Psychoanalytic Inquiry: A Topical Journal for Mental Health Professionals*, the Psychoanalytic Inquiry Book Series presents a diversity of subjects within a diversity of approaches to those subjects. Under the editorship of Joseph Lichtenberg, in collaboration with Melvin Bornstein and the editorial board of *Psychoanalytic Inquiry*, the volumes in this series strike a balance between research, theory, and clinical application. We are honored to have published the works of various innovators in psychoanalysis, including Frank Lachmann, James Fosshage, Robert Stolorow, Donna Orange, Louis Sander, Léon Wurmser, James Grotstein, Joseph Jones, Doris Brothers, Fredric Busch, and Joseph Lichtenberg, among others.

The series includes books and monographs on mainline psychoanalytic topics, such as sexuality, narcissism, trauma, homosexuality, jealousy, envy, and varied aspects of analytic process and technique. In our efforts to broaden the field of analytic interest, the series has incorporated and embraced innovative discoveries in infant research, self psychology, intersubjectivity, motivational systems, affects as process, responses to cancer, borderline states, contextualism, postmodernism, attachment research and theory, medication, and mentalization. As further investigations in psychoanalysis come to fruition, we seek to present them in readable, easily comprehensible writing.

After more than 25 years, the core vision of this series remains the investigation, analysis and discussion of developments on the cutting edge of the psychoanalytic field, inspired by a boundless spirit of inquiry. A full list of all the titles available in the *Psychoanalytic Inquiry* Book Series is available at https://www.routledge.com/Psychoanalytic-Inquiry-Book- Series/book-series/LEAPIBS.

THE PSYCHOANALYTIC ZERO

A Decolonizing Study of Therapeutic Dialogues

Koichi Togashi

Routledge
Taylor & Francis Group
LONDON AND NEW YORK

First published 2020
by Routledge
2 Park Square, Milton Park, Abingdon, Oxon OX14 4RN

and by Routledge
52 Vanderbilt Avenue, New York, NY 10017

Routledge is an imprint of the Taylor & Francis Group, an informa business

British Library Cataloguing-in-Publication Data
A catalogue record for this book is available from the British Library

Library of Congress Cataloging-in-Publication Data
Names: Togashi, Koichi (Psychoanalyst), author.
Title: The psychoanalytic zero : a decolonizing study of
therapeutic dialogues / Koichi Togashi.
Description: Abingdon, Oxon ; New York, NY : Routledge, 2020.
Identifiers: LCCN 2019046197 (print) | LCCN 2019046198 (ebook) |
ISBN 9780367859350 (hardback) | ISBN 9780367859374 (paperback) |
ISBN 9781003015871 (ebook)
Subjects: LCSH: Psychoanalysis. | Psychotherapy.
Classification: LCC RC506 .T64 2020 (print) | LCC RC506 (ebook) |
DDC 616.89/17--dc23
LC record available at https://lccn.loc.gov/2019046197
LC ebook record available at https://lccn.loc.gov/2019046198

ISBN: 978-0-367-85935-0 (hbk)
ISBN: 978-0-367-85937-4 (pbk)
ISBN: 978-1-003-01587-1 (ebk)

Typeset in Bembo
by Taylor & Francis Books

CONTENTS

FIGURE

PREFACE

A professional psychoanalytic encounter begins with a therapist explaining the professional service she can provide for her patient. Alternatively, it starts when the therapist begins to collect information in order to diagnose the patient. Or it may commence with the therapist simply attempting to empathically listen to the patient. Any and all of these professional proceedings, however, occur only *after* the two people have a *human* encounter.

You receive a phone-call from a person who seeks help. You hear the voice and respond to it, not because the person is a patient, but because he or she is human. Even if the call is a wrong number, intended for someone else, there is still a response and engagement with the person that precedes awareness of the patient, a response before there is any sense of the person's anguish, shame, loneliness, anger, or sadness; and before you are aware of your own role or meaning. There is a response that precedes any positive or negative feelings toward the person, any sense of liking or feeling sorry for them, that precedes any experience of kinship or even the bare business relationship of customer and provider. This is the moment without context, in which the person who exists in your presence is merely another human being.

Being precedes awareness. At this moment without context, you are not yet a "therapist;" the person you are speaking to is not yet a "patient." This is the moment in which a psychoanalytic world is born and within it, the roles of patient and therapist. At this moment, the context is created between you and the person you are engaged with, and both of you are aware who you are within this context.

There are no procedures being enacted at the initial moment of being. Once in the professional setting, the patient may dissolve into tears, talk in an emotionless manner, or become irritated. The therapist who observes the patient's actions characterizes him or her as "narcissistic," "traumatized," "pathological," or sees the patient as a person who does not have sufficient reality testing to make a professional contract. No matter what the assessment is, the result is inevitably to make one person more of a *patient*, and the other more a *therapist*. These correspondences are born out of their initial encounter, and the nature of the encounter is born out of these roles.

Context is born out of a moment without context. The moment of encounter between a person who comes to be called a patient and a person who comes to be called a therapist is the zero moment of psychoanalysis. Once the context is defined as psychoanalytic work, however, those same people, *who simply existed at the zero moment*, are immediately objectified with certain roles and forms, namely, "a patient with pain" and "a therapist with a professional role." Yet we persist in the illusion that the *patient* and the *therapist* have always been there.

Picture in your mind a "love-starved" patient, or a "hostile" patient. Does the person with the diagnosis exist before the therapist encounters them? Does a "business-like therapist" or an "authoritarian therapist" exist before meeting the patient? Typically, the clinician thinks of the patient as inherently love-starved or hostile but believes that she herself is neutral until the appropriate therapeutic stance is called for in response. For the clinician, the world exists in a certain form before she is aware of herself, and she judges it only afterward.

Such an attitude imposes a cost in terms of humanness. The person in your presence becomes an abstracted object called a *patient*; and you become another abstracted object, a professional role called *therapist*. This perspective gives both parties a sense of certainty; for the person named as a patient-object, you are identified as a psychoanalytic professional, and your encounter with the *person* is defined as professional work. But once these roles are named, the relationship loses a flexible ambiguity and is caught in a world retroactively contextualized through *Nachträglichkeit*, or "making sense backward." Evaluation—*naming*—gives you and your patient a worldview that is felt as accurate and certain, but narrowed. The contextualized world makes many aspects of a human encounter invisible, and often denies them outright. Still, as clinicians, we cannot resist the temptation.

The moment without context exists not only at the very first encounter, but also *in every moment* of psychoanalytic work from a whole session to a ten-year analysis. A therapeutic dialogue, therefore, can be seen as a succession of context-free moments, inclusive of every possibility and continually creating context, moment by moment. But unless we are aware of it, the moment becomes invisible, hidden within the context that the moment itself creates.

The *psychoanalytic zero* is a perspective that includes awareness of the moment without context and calls for clinicians to embrace its possibilities and surrender themselves to the primal moment of human encounter in our clinical practice.

As professionals, we meet each new patient with a perspective encumbered with psychoanalytic theories, procedures, our experience of the human mind and body, society and culture. Still, at the very moment of human encounter none of these perspectives apply, and the world that we and our patients will create does not yet exist.

Once we are aware of this *reversal of recognition*, we can see the zero everywhere in our long-term therapeutic work. We often have moments in which we are just *being* with our patients, staying in the moment with no thought about our therapeutic roles, theories, or formality. While the zero point is not the embodiment of a mental state, one's mental state *can be* an expression of an analyst's *surrendering* to emptiness. All the moments of a therapeutic session cannot be planned, and prepared. Presence coexists with absence, and these spare moments offer the possibility of recreating the original human encounter, the infinite space from which the therapeutic dyad can be born.

The psychoanalytic zero and the Eastern perspective

The psychoanalytic zero is neither a temporal point nor a spatial structure, but an aspect of Nature emerging in analytic work from which everything is born and to which everything is reduced. The zero point does not connote absence or non-presence but means nothing and everything. This idea has its roots in East Asian culture in which value systems, despite some difference in historical development, typically include the philosophy of emptiness or nothingness (Lopez, 1998; Ai, 2006; Møllgaard, 2007). The Eastern concept of emptiness and nothingness are both often mistakenly understood as a culturally unique concept of a boundary-less relationship between people, or something akin to the concept of "we-self" (Moore, 1983; Roland, 1996), but it is inherently different, for the notion of "we-self" includes, a priori, the idea of the division between self, other, and we as a group.

Emptiness or nothingness is grounded in a nameless and concept-less universe in which there are no distinctions between any named entities of the world; no distinction between self, other, and we, nor any bonding between them. In the concept-less universe, there is neither presence nor absence. I am we and the other, and the other is me and we. Naming creates division, discrimination, and injustice in the world. In other words, naming creates a wounded world, the traumatized world.

In Buddhist tradition, the idea of *Sunyata*, emptiness, is considered to have been first propounded by Nagarjuna in the 2nd or 3rd Century CE, and has been carried over into other Buddhist sects, including Zen Buddhism in Japan. This idea was systematically organized in the well-known Mahayana Buddhist writing, the Heart Sutra. The Heart Sutra discourses on the "wisdom" of Buddhism, the insight into the true nature of the universe, which is impermanence, suffering, non-self, and emptiness. The Heart Sutra famously expresses the philosophy of emptiness as, "Form is exactly emptiness, emptiness is exactly form." Emptiness is not separate from form, form is not separate from emptiness. Whatever is form is emptiness, whatever is emptiness is form.

Taoism (Daoism),[1] a philosophical tradition of Chinese origin, teaches the existence of *Tao*, the Way, a transcendent principle of the universe. In the *Taoist* philosophy of nothingness, Nature is a dynamically continuous flow, infinitely changing and moving, and involving all aspects of being in the universe. This is the universe that has neither concepts nor names. There are no distinctions and all contradictions are resolved. Absence does not mean non-presence, but rather, absence *is* presence. *Taoists*, despite differences between particular schools, generally emphasize effortless action, "naturalness" and "spontaneity," which entails surrender to Nature. *Taoism* differs from Buddhism and Confucianism, but each has influenced the other. *Tao,* the central tenet of *Taoism*, is often seen as a fundamental principle in many East Asian philosophical schools (Ai, 2006; Møllgaard, 2007).

Makoto is a metaphysical principle in which personal will or agency is renounced, drawing human beings and Nature together in the same current, a tide which is not contaminated by any human thoughts or artificial controls. Many Japanese philosophers (Ishikawa, 1938; Watsuji, 1952; Sagara, 1980, 1998a, 1998b; Shimokawa, 2001) recognized that the essence of this moral philosophy has become deeply embedded in many aspects of Japanese culture, including political attitudes, economic activities, education and others. The *makoto* form of Japanese ethics has its origins in the ancient Shinto idea of *seimei-shin* (purity in mind) (Watsuji, 1952). This principle evolved into the more explicitly moral value, *makoto* or "*shisei*," in the early modern period, influenced by Neo-Confucian moral values of the Wang Yang-Ming school in the Edo era (1603–1868). The fundamental ethic of *makoto* is not found in an objective norm or order, but in an attitude and pursuit of selflessness and purity of sentiment. It is not merely a sincere state of mind but a reflection of the cosmic tide of Nature, ever transforming and changing.

The concept of emptiness, which forms the theoretical background of the psychoanalytic zero, is inherently different from the basic principles that run through most psychoanalytic writings. As many recent writers have noted, traditional psychoanalytic theories embrace dichotomies such as mind versus body, self versus other, presence versus absence, etc. (see for example, Frie, 1997; Stolorow, Atwood, and Orange, 2002; Stolorow, 2011b). But, as my colleague and I maintain (Brothers and Togashi, 2019), even recent psychoanalytic perspectives that are critical of these Cartesian dichotomies remain within the Western values that presuppose conceptual divisions in the human world. In traditional psychoanalytic writings, presence does not mean absence, and self does not mean the other. The *psychoanalytic zero,* in this sense, is a new perspective that seeks to enrich the dimensions of an analytic relationship, and to contribute to the decolonization of psychoanalysis.

The effort of decolonizing traditional psychoanalytic perspectives is one of finding alternative ways of thinking that serve to decenter the cultural, social, and economic capital of Western paternalism. As psychoanalysts, we are inevitably laden with prejudices—embedded through our personal development in a certain culture and professional development in a certain psychoanalytic training—that tend to make us blind in our understanding of the therapeutic process, as well as in our understanding of the world, as discussed previously. In this book, the reader may have to put aside familiar ways of thinking and responding, based on assumptions baked into standard psychoanalytic literature and practice, in order to encounter the very different and unfamiliar conceptions of emptiness and zero. It is not my intention to create new theories or replace existing ideas, but simply to introduce a different way of thinking and to conceptualize a kind of experience and practice. This book will try to illustrate how this new perspective sheds light on our therapeutic practice and will offer a new way of understanding human suffering.

The concept of the psychoanalytic zero broadens our mental horizons in clinical practice. The moment without context unfolds in an intersubjective field that is beyond the integrity or unity of an individual mind, a field that is continually transforming and changing. The patient and analyst whose minds remain open to reflect the tide of the intersubjective field are subject to, and become part of, the principle of Nature. The psychoanalytic zero may require a letting go of personal values and thoughts, or a relinquishing of social and professional roles. It is just these definable forms and roles that produce clinical phenomena such as transference, countertransference, co-transference, resistance, or enactment, all of which may or may not produce suffering for our patients.

From the Eastern ethical perspective, human suffering is created by one's preoccupation with naming observed phenomenon, including the distinction between oneself and the other. From this point of view, trauma is neither a human experience nor an actual event but an emergent worldview. Trauma is the beginning of the need for names, and naming the world creates all human experiences, including anguish and suffering, happiness and well-being. Indeed, in this model, anguish and suffering are no different from happiness and well-being. Trauma makes a person aware of the wounded nature of the world and awakens this awareness with powerful emotional impact. Without trauma, people would not be able to see the world, including themselves and others.

Content outline

This book consists of two parts: Part I: Emptiness and the psychoanalytic zero, which covers Chapters 1 through 5, discusses how the psychoanalytic zero lends a new perspective to the analytic relationship. Part II: Human suffering and the experience of being human, consisting of Chapters 6 through 9, explores how we might understand and approach human suffering and anguish through this new perspective.

The first chapter, "Surrender and silence: The problem of narrative and non-narrative in psychoanalysis," focuses on two ideas: Ghent's (1990) concept of surrender, and narrative. Making use of my own cultural background, I attempt to relate Ghent's surrender to emptiness, a traditional Eastern ethical value.

Chapter 2, "Beyond the guilt of being: Surrender to emptiness," proposes an Asian perspective on the "ethical turn" in psychoanalysis through analytic work with a patient who feels guilt about her being. In working through this suffering, the analyst and patient are required to surrender themselves to emptiness, creating a space before or beyond right and wrong or good and bad.

Chapter 3 is entitled "An Asian ethical perspective on sincerity in psychoanalysis." Many Japanese philosophers and ethicists have drawn attention to the cultural idiosyncrasies of *makoto*, one of the essential aspects of Japanese ethics. In this chapter, I review the intersubjective process by which *makoto* emerges between a patient and an analyst. In this example, I argue that a relational purity, rather than the therapist's consistent behavior, was the proper focus of both participants' efforts.

Chapter 4, entitled "The motivational system of moving toward zero," explores the meaning of silence and emptiness in the light of motivational systems theory and attempts to illustrate the psychoanalytic zero within a Western psychoanalytic model.

Chapter 5, "Trauma, contingency, and the psychoanalytic zero," begins the examination of suffering and its relation to the experience of being human. Trauma is neither an experience nor an actual event, but the beginning of the "human" condition. The argument is illustrated through interwoven narratives of transgenerational trauma that arose in the psychoanalytic treatment of a traumatized patient whose parents were atomic bomb survivors in Hiroshima and Nagasaki. It describes the patient's and analyst's surrender to the nameless universe in which the division between victim and victimizer is a production of contingency.

Chapter 6, "Being thrown into the world without informed consent," discusses how a traumatic event strikes a person without their knowledge, willing agreement, or permission. In a review of the case vignette of a female patient suffering from complex trauma, the relation of informed consent to traumatic events is seen as a form of existential anguish, a response to living in a contemporary world of contingency. I argue that the lack of informed consent to a traumatic event can violate one's sense of responsibility, and go on to show how we may undertake the process of granting informed consent retrospectively in a therapeutic process.

Chapter 7 is titled "From traumatized individuality to being human with others: Intersubjective taboo and unspoken reality." Traumatized patients often experience themselves as being alienated from human society. Using the perspective of a decolonizing study of therapeutic dialogues, I attempt to illustrate a dyadic process that may transform the patient's alienation into a sense of being human with others.

Chapter 8, "A sense of 'being human' and twinship experience," illustrates the ways in which a person experiences himself or herself as being human, including being treated as human by others. This study consists of a review of the literature in clinical ethics and psychoanalysis, and psycho-biographical research on Heinz Kohut, who sought the meaning of being human while in the grip of a ten-year struggle with lymphoma.

In the final chapter, "The problem of uncertainty: The future of psychoanalysis," I discuss how the division between certainty and uncertainty is an artificial human construct that emerges in a traumatized world. Through a case vignette with a Japanese patient, I show how the psychoanalytic zero requires the analyst to surrender him or herself to the moment without division between certainty and uncertainty.

A note on "language-games"

The Psychoanalytic Zero: A Decolonizing Study of Therapeutic Dialogues is my second book written in English. Writing a book is always challenging but writing a book in a second language is particularly demanding, and at the same time fascinating and thrilling. While preparing this book, I have experienced moments in which two kinds of "language-games" (Wittgenstein, 1953) encounter each other. The "rules" for an English word highlight potential meanings in an equivalent Japanese word, which reflects new implications onto the original English and, occasionally, sheds new light on hidden aspects of both. In the process, I have had the good fortune to find new understandings of both the human world and the psychoanalytic world.

Although I have had this experience with every English language paper I've written, the language-games have played out with particular resonance in this book, because it takes as its subject the decolonization of psychoanalytic dialogue. In every chapter—almost every paragraph—Western and Eastern language and concepts meet, converse, and struggle to understand each other. Readers may feel some disorientation from this back and forth, but I hope they can enjoy the play between two languages and cultures and, ultimately, join in the game.

Note

1 The two words, *Tao* and *Dao, Taoism* and *Daoism*, have been used interchangeably in English. In this book, I use "*Tao*" and "*Taoism*" because *Dao* has a different meaning in Confucianism, related to moral principles and rules of one's social role in society. I am grateful to a friend and colleague, Liling Lin, MSW for explaining to me the basic difference between them. (Lin, 2018, personal communication).

ACKNOWLEDGEMENTS

I would like to acknowledge those who have provided significant support for me to make this language match possible. I express my deep gratitude, first and foremost, to Dr. Roger Frie for his encouragement and guidance during the writing of this book, particularly the original articles that have become Chapters 1 and 8, and, of course, for our personal friendship. I am also grateful to special colleagues and friends Doris Brothers, Ph.D., Joseph D. Lichtenberg, M.D., Margy Sperry, Ph.D., Maxwell S. Sucharov, M.D., and Donna M. Orange, Ph.D., Psy.D. for their careful reading and productive critiques of the original articles for each chapter, and to my personal editor, Mort Milder, for his careful editing and thoughtful suggestions for making my English voice more English and yet still recognizably my own.

I am also grateful to my patients who have given me the great opportunity and privilege of sharing their lives in my offices. I thank those who come from the psychoanalytic communities in the United States, Taiwan, and Japan, and who have stimulated me and inspired my thinking in many ways. I wish to express my gratitude to Arthur A. Gray, Ph.D., Amy Joelson, M.S.W., Amanda Kottler, M.A., Frank M. Lachmann, Ph.D., Elizabeth F. Feldman, Jackie Gotthold, Psy.D., Shelley R. Doctors, Ph.D., Beatrice Beebe, Ph.D., Jeffrey Stern, Ph.D., Jessica Benjamin, Ph.D., Jill Gentile, Ph.D., James L. Fosshage, Ph.D., Jill R. Gardner, Ph.D., George Hagman, C.S.W, L.C.S.W., Peter Kaufmann, Ph.D., Catherine Hicks, Ph. D., Estelle Shane, Ph.D., and Peter B. Zimmermann in the Western community, mainly the United States; to Soh Agatsuma, M.D., Ph.D., Ken Okano, M.D., Ph. D., Koichi Yokoi, M.D., Kosuke Tsuiki, Ph.D., Makiko Kasai, Ph.D., Kazunori Nakanishi, M.A., Naoki Fujiyama, M.D., Ph.D., Osamu Fukumoto, M.D., Ph.D., Michie Harada, M.A., and Naoki Yasumura, M.A. in Japan; and Hao-Chung Hsu, M.D., Kelly Chang, M.D., Hui-Ching Liu, M.D., Sileng Lau, M.D., Hsiu-Hui Huang, M.A., and Liling Lin, M.S.W in Taiwan, for their long-term friendship and reading of my works, and for the many ways in which they have encouraged my aspirations for this long-term exploration.

Finally, I thank Routledge, Ms. Kate Hawes, Ms. Hannah Wright, and the other production editors for giving me the opportunity of publishing this book and helping my work throughout its production.

Parts of this book originally appeared as individual articles or presentations at conferences, as indicated below, though revised for this publication. I would like to officially acknowledge Taylor and Francis for permitting the reprinting of Chapters 1, 6, 8, and a part of Epilogue. Furthermore, I would like to acknowledge Pro-Ed Publishing Company for kindly permitting the reprinting of Chapter 9.

Chapter 8, "A sense of 'being human' and twinship experience" is funded by a grant from the Uehiro Foundation on Ethics and Education, Tokyo, Japan, and is dedicated to Dr. Toshihiko Maruta.

Chapter 1: (2019). "Surrender and silence: The problem of narrative and non-narrative in psychoanalysis narrative as the zero." *Psychoanalysis, Self and Context*, published online.

Chapter 2: (2017). "Beyond the guilt of being: Surrender to the psychoanalytic zero." Original paper presented at the 14th Conference on the International Association for Relational Psychoanalysis & Psychotherapy, Sydney, Australia.

Chapter 3: (2017). "An Asian ethical perspective on sincerity in psychoanalysis." Original paper presented at the Psychology & the Other Conference, 2017, Boston, MA.

Chapter 4: (2016). "The motivational system of moving toward nothingness." Original paper presented at the 2016 Taiwan Self Psychology Conference, Taipei, Taiwan.

Chapter 5: (2019). "Trauma, contingency and the psychoanalytic zero." Original paper presented at the 42nd Annual International Conference on the Psychology of the Self, Vancouver, Canada.

Chapter 6: (2017). "Being thrown into the world without informed consent." *Psychoanalysis, Self and Context*, 12(1), 20–34.

Chapter 7: (2016). "From traumatized individuality to being human with others: Intersubjective taboo and unspoken reality." Paper presented at the 39th Annual International Conference on the Psychology of the Self, Boston, MA.

Chapter 8: (2014). "A sense of "being human" and twinship experience." *International Journal of Psychoanalytic Self Psychology*, 9(4), 265–281.

Chapter 9: (2015). "The value of living with uncertainty and its relevance for analytic work." *Podium of Psychoanalysis: Self Psychology*, 12 & 13 (pp. 279-,294), Taipei, Taiwan: Pro-Ed Publishing Company.

Epilogue: (2010). "An effort to find self psychological concepts in an Asian culture." *International Journal of Psychoanalytic Self Psychology*, 5(1), 113–115.

PART I

Emptiness and the psychoanalytic zero

1

SURRENDER AND SILENCE

The problem of narrative and non-narrative in psychoanalysis

Psychoanalytic work most often occurs through narrative. The patient describes his or her experience in narrative form, attempting to create order out of chaos (Murray, 2003) and using narrative as an organizing principle (Sarbin, 1986). The analyst listens to the narrative and pieces together scraps of information of all sorts from the patient's account of his or her daily life. The patient and analyst observe and attach meaning to these scraps, and then create stories with spatially structured and temporally consistent plots. I would like to suggest, however, that the analyst's preoccupation with theoretical models and formulation of a psychoanalytic narrative can be limiting as well as liberating. By examining the uses of surrender, Nature, and emptiness in relation to narrative, I believe we can expand the possibilities in the psychoanalytic dyad.

Surrender, East and West

Emmanuel Ghent's (1990) innovative and pioneering idea of "surrender" is widely accepted and praised by contemporary psychoanalysts, especially in the intersubjective and relational schools. By distinguishing "surrender" from "submission," Ghent makes clear that surrender need not imply "defeat" or "giving in to the other," but may be "a quality of liberation and 'letting-go'" (p.118). While submission is a relational form in which a submissive individual is subjected to a dominant other, and the submissive's identity, sense of self, and sense of wholeness atrophy, surrender involves the "discovery of one's identity, one's sense of self, one's sense of wholeness, even one's sense of unity with other living beings" (p. 111). Ghent emphasizes that in Eastern philosophies, the term "surrender" is associated with transcendence and liberation.

Despite some differences of emphasis, contemporary psychoanalytic thinkers (Aron, 2005; Benjamin, 2004, 2007, 2018; Orange, 2008, 2011; Togashi, 2017c, 2017g;

Knoblauch, 2018) all advance the view that surrender plays an important role in the psychoanalytic process, that it implies freedom from any interest to control or dominate, as well as a devotion to human relationships, and allows for creativity and development to unfold in the intersubjective field. They emphasize that surrender is often necessary to break an impasse or repetitive loop in the therapeutic process.

Benjamin (2004, 2007, 2018) emphasizes that surrender need not be to someone, in a one-way fashion, but may be to a space of thirdness. She maintains that "the Third" is the position from which a patient and analyst can recognize each other as having a shared subject yet experience each other as individual minds. She writes that "the Third refers to the position constituted through holding the tension of recognition between sameness and difference, taking the other to be a separate but equivalent center of initiative and consciousness with whom nonetheless feelings and intentions can be shared" (Benjamin, 2018, p.4). When an analytic relationship gets caught in a "complementary" dynamic (Benjamin, 1990), in which each partner feels that his or her perspective is the only right one, an analyst's (and a patient's) surrendering to the Third helps them achieve mutual recognition, the ability to let go of a certain part of the self and take in the other's perspective.

Orange (2011) understands Ghent's *surrender* as resembling Levinasian passivity or receptivity. In her "hermeneutics of trust" (Orange, 2011), she describes the psychoanalytic process as radically asymmetrical and an analyst as primarily a respondent to the patients' suffering. For Orange, this ethical response precedes an analyst's recognition of her own subjectivity or willingness. She argues that an analyst cannot resist feeling concern and responding once she has seen the suffering face of her patient, and casts herself into infinite responsibility to him. In this ethic, an analyst's surrendering to the patient is no longer agentic or chosen. For Orange, unlike Benjamin (2007, 2018), surrender is not to the field or a position, but to the Other, or the call for responsibility from the Other. This ethical response precedes an analyst's recognition of her own subjectivity or willingness.

Although these are useful insights—courageous efforts to adapt Ghent's ideas to contemporary psychoanalysis—Benjamin and Orange's conceptions of surrender are still grounded in a Western perspective. Their models view analytic fields as organized between two subjectivities, even when they assume the third, or ethical, field in which both participants escape from the subject-other distinction. Ghent's innovative contribution, however, draws on his understanding of Buddhism and his special interest in Eastern philosophies. He sees the concept of surrender in relation to "'*emptiness*,' the beneficent state of being that is at the center of the *Tao* [*Dao*]" (Ghent, 1990, p.113; emphasis added), and adds that surrender can be expressed in many forms depending on culture Ghent (1990) states:

> My hunch is that there is something like a universal need, wish or longing for what I am calling surrender and that it assumes many forms. In some societies there are culturally sanctioned occasions for its realization in the form of ecstatic rituals and healing trances. In other societies, perhaps most notably in Japan where the psychology of *amae* is so central to one's way of being,

> something akin to surrender is experienced as almost universally desired and desirable. In many people in our own culture the wish for surrender remains buried; in some it is expressed in creative and productive ways, and in others its derivatives appear in pathological form, deflected away from normal channels by that most unwelcome price-tag: dread. I suspect further that this dread is something that we have encountered in other contexts and have conceptualized as annihilation anxiety, dread of dissolution, ego fragmentation and so on.
>
> *(Ghent, 1990, p.114)*

For Ghent, surrender is transcendence of the fear of death or annihilation. In the transcendence of this fear, one commits him or herself to an experience which could shatter his or her belief system and threaten a sense of being. It is only in the transcendence of the painful contemplation of non-existence, Ghent (1990) states, that one can reach radical emptiness in one's personal or relational development and obtain a new sense of unity or relief in the presence of other living beings. He emphasizes that surrender is neither to a person nor a space, nor ethical responses nor actions. He says that "one cannot choose to surrender. … One can provide facilitative conditions for surrender but cannot make it happen" (Ghent, 1990, p.109).

Taoism or *Daoism*, the ideological background of Ghent's concept of surrender, is "an ancient legacy of the East Asian culture" (Ai, 2006, p.149). It is more a cosmology than a religion or psychology. It presupposes neither the existence of an afterlife nor a benevolent divinity but, instead, is premised on the idea of an unintentional principle of Nature that precedes and underlies all of reality. *Tao*, which refers to "the way" or "universal principle" in Chinese tradition, implies this ultimate, indefinable principle underlying all movements (Møllgaard, 2007); a fundamental dynamic principle that also exists *within* all things. The founder of *Taoism*, Lao Zi, states in the first chapter of his scripture, *The Tao Te Ching*:

> Chapter 1 THE EMBODIMENT OF TAO
>
> Even the finest teaching is not the Tao itself.
> Even the finest name is insufficient to define it.
> Without words, the Tao can be experienced,
> and without a name, it can be known.
>
> To conduct one's life according to the Tao,
> is to conduct one's life without regrets;
> to realize that potential within oneself
> which is of benefit to all.
>
> Though words or names are not required
> to live one's life this way,
> to describe it, words and names are used,
> that we might better clarify

the way of which we speak,
without confusing it with other ways
in which an individual might choose to live.

Through knowledge, intellectual thought and words,
the manifestations of the Tao are known,
but without such intellectual intent
we might experience the Tao itself.

Both knowledge and experience are real,
but reality has many forms,
which seem to cause complexity.

By using the means appropriate,
we extend ourselves beyond
the barriers of such complexity,
and so experience the Tao.

(Translated by Rosenthal, from National Taiwan University Library, 2018)

Lao Zi emphasizes that *Tao* is the indefinable and *nameless* universe infinitely changing and moving. In our "human" world, which has a need for names, *Tao* is divided and dichotomies emerge. "Not big" means "small," "not ugly" means "beautiful," and so on. Such is the human condition, the artificial "world that results in the neglect of the world qua world" (Møllgaard, 2007, p.17). But in the indefinable and nameless universe, there are no dichotomies, and all contradictions coexist. "Not poor" does not mean wealthy, "not good" does not mean "bad." In this universe, presence is absence and absence is presence. If presence disappears, absence does not take its place, but also disappears. Lao Zi emphasizes this basic principle of Nature and recommends that people surrender themselves to it. He states:

Chapter 5 WITHOUT INTENTION

Nature acts without intent,
so cannot be described
as acting with benevolence,
nor malevolence to any thing.

In this respect, the Tao is just the same,
though in reality it should be said
that nature follows the rule of Tao.

Therefore, even when he seems to act
in manner kind or benevolent,
the sage is not acting with such intent,
for in conscious matters such as these,
he is amoral and indifferent.

The sage retains tranquility,
and is not by speech or thought disturbed,
and even less by action which is contrived.
His actions are spontaneous,
as are his deeds towards his fellow men.

By this means he is empty of desire,
and his energy is not drained from him.
(Translated by Rosenthal, from National Taiwan University Library, 2018)

Lao Zi's poetic description suggests that in the original idea of *Taoism*, surrender is neither to the third place between two entities nor to the ethical response to the other. Instead, surrender is to Nature, the nameless universe, or what Ghent calls *emptiness.*

For Ghent, what we surrender tois not the painful and meaningless *emptiness* people may imagine and, in order to proceed, the reader is asked to put aside some assumptions derived from standard psychoanalytic literature and practice, and encounter what is perhaps a very different and unfamiliar conception of emptiness. *Taoism*'s Nature, or Ghent's emptiness is the moment without context, in which neither a sense of being, a living experience, nor a meeting of the other has yet emerged. It is the moment that is not defined by personal will or agency, or determined by human thought or artificial control. To borrow a convenient metaphor from physics, it is a black hole, to which everything is reduced and from which everything comes.

As an example of his notion of surrender, which aligns with an "Eastern sensibility," Ghent (1990) refers to Zen satori. Zen Buddhism derives from a different historical background than *Taoism,* yet satori—awareness of the essence of the universe—is a closely related concept. The Heart Sutra, one of the central scriptures of Zen Buddhism, preaches that the essence of the universe is absolute emptiness, as well as its negation, encapsulated in the famous phrase, "Form is exactly emptiness, emptiness is exactly form." This implies that all being in the universe is insubstantial and intangible. Also implied in this phrase is the suspension of all artificial categorizations, such as you/me, subject/object, and inside/outside.

Many Eastern philosophers (Watsuji, 1952; Nishida, 1958; Sagara, 1980, 1998b; Abe & Heine, 1992; Møllgaard, 2007) maintain that the concept of emptiness has strongly influenced many fields of East Asian culture and is inherent in people's thoughts and habits. In this conception, all beings and entities in this world are seen as a part of an indefinable Nature, and there are no self/other differences. It should be noted that this is not like the "we-self" quality that has been discussed by some Western theorists (Moore, 1983; Roland, 1996). There are not even differences between the individual and "we."

How is the therapeutic dyad altered in the face of this absolute emptiness? It is suggested that the therapist (and often the patient) go through a process of surrendering themselves. But how is this process of surrender to be understood?

Psychoanalysis often uses narrative to make sense of the therapeutic process (Searles, 1965), to put the ineffable into words and to find a way of telling stories that are waiting to be heard (Freeman, 2002, 2012; Frie, 2012a, 2016). A personal experience is organized through narration of a story. This personal experience is always already embedded in relational, cultural, and historical contexts, which can include elements that the narrator is not even aware of. Contemporary relational psychoanalytic and narrative thinkers (Cushman 1995, 2011; Freeman, 2002, 2012; Frie, 2012a, 2016) no longer limit narrative to the spoken revelation of personal stories and memories but conceptualize it to include untold and unthought stories as well. These narrative perspectives implicitly include elements that are closely related to surrender and emptiness.

Freeman (2012) advocates the idea of

> the narrative unconscious in reference to those culturally rooted aspects of one's history that have not yet become part of one's story. They are hidden, not so much in the sense of that which has been buried through the forceful work of repression as that which remains unthought and is, therefore, not yet a part of the story I can tell.
>
> *(Freeman, 2012, p. 362)*

These contributions expand the idea of narrative, but do not allow for the idea of emptiness in itself; they still conceptualize what is unspoken as an expression of something that has been disavowed, unformulated, or remains unorganized. Similarly, for relational theorists, *dissociation* presupposes that there is something that is sequestered (Bromberg, 2009), and *unformulated experience* presupposes that there is something to be formulated (Stern, 2010). Neither notion includes the existence of emptiness as Eastern philosophy characterizes it. It may be that the "surrender to emptiness" lies outside the use of narrative in relational psychoanalysis; in other words, we have to ask if it is always the case that there are stories, told or untold, in the analytic dialogue, or can we be open to our patient's accounts without formulating stories about it? Might the analyst's preoccupation with formulating a narrative, in fact, limit his or her vision? In posing this question, my aim is not to displace an existing concept of surrender. Rather, I want employ my cultural background to expand the discussion with an alternative conception that may be unfamiliar to Western trained psychoanalysts—and I do not exclude myself, because my psychoanalytic training was also in the West.

Non-narrative in psychoanalysis

Psychoanalysis has paid attention to a patient's action of not narrating. Through the idea of resistance, Freud (1896) provides a procedure to work through a patient's failure or inability to talk fully about his or her subjective experience. This is based on the premise that there are unarticulated psychic processes in a patient's mind.

Freud's (1900–01) idea of the unconscious refers to a topographical space in the mind which consists of what is not narrated and what is not organized enough to be narrated.

Using this model, Freud understood an analyst's job to be the discovery of truth in two senses. Freud (Breuer & Freud, 1893) originally saw psychoanalytic practice as a way to find a "true event" in the past that was missing from a patient's memory. Later, he came to believe that the recovered memory was not necessarily of a real event (Freud, 1925b) and saw analysis as a way to identify an etiological fantasy in the unconscious that could complete the patient's non-narrative. Either way, for Freud, psychoanalysis is an archaeological project in which the purpose is to uncover a hidden past.

Spence (1982), however, criticizes this premise in Freudian psychoanalysis. For him, an analyst's work is not to find or discover something which has been buried in the depths of the unconscious. It is a project in which an analyst and a patient weave a story with the most plausible plot by pulling together pieces of memories, fantasies, and associations. In this perspective, meanings are not discovered in narrative and non-narrative; they are produced by both participants.

Schafer (1983, 1992) also criticizes the Freudian view of the analyst as an authority who knows the one correct story in and behind a patient's non-narrative. Schafer, like Spence, emphasizes that psychoanalysis is not a practice that digs out a true, but hidden, story, but a practice that co-authors a story about a patient's non-narrated anguished life. The analyst, in this perspective, is a professional who reformulates a patient's non-narrative and retells a story that both participants make sense of together. Schafer (1983) states:

> People going through psychoanalysis—analysands—tell the analyst about themselves and others in the past and present. In making interpretations, the analyst retells these stories. In the retelling, certain features are accentuated while others are placed in parentheses; certain features are related to others in new ways or for the first time; some features are developed further, perhaps at great length. This retelling is done along psychoanalytic lines ... The analyst's retellings progressively influence the what and how of the stories told by analysands. The analyst establishes new, though often contested or resisted, questions that amount to regulated narrative possibilities. The end product of this interweaving of texts is a radically new, jointly authored work or way of working.
>
> *(Schafer, 1983, p.219)*

Schafer's paradigm shift to a hermeneutic constructivist vision is not only drastically opposed to the classical ideal of scientific objectivity in Freudian psychoanalysis, but also illustrates the transformational power of narrative to reshape a patient's life. There are two significant implications of this approach to narrative for psychoanalysis: first, narrative is always and already situated in the personal, cultural, and historical context; second, narrative includes cultural and historical elements that "are often disclosed through language in ways that we are not even aware of" (Frie, 2012a, p.331). The constructivist view frees the analyst from the limiting belief that there is one and only one truth, thus suggesting that truth is "co-constructed." The analyst proceeds with the expectation that he will co-construct a story with his patient that might make sense of the state of a patient's mind.

Despite their manifest differences, the models of Freud and Schafer both assume the existence of a feasible story, and rely on the belief that the analyst can reconstruct or re-author a story in and behind the patient's narrative. As such, neither perspective includes the notion of emptiness. There are always separate but related aspects involved: spoken and unspoken, telling and not-telling.

A similar observation can be made of recent discussions of non-narrative and trauma. Herman (1992), in her innovative study of trauma, describes the process by which victims lose the ability to relate traumatic memories through verbal narrative: "Traumatic memories lack verbal narrative and context; rather, they are encoded in the form of vivid sensations and images" (Herman, 1992, p.38). For her, traumatic memories are no longer encoded in ordinary verbal form; they do not become linear narratives that are easily assimilated into an ongoing life story, but take the form of an "idee fixe," which "breaks spontaneously into consciousness, both as flashbacks during waking states and as traumatic nightmares during sleep" (p.38).

Following Herman, Caruth (1996) sees a complex connection between traumatic memory, non-narrative, and re-enactment. She argues that trauma is not experienced until it is re-experienced, stressing the repetitive nature in the form of enactment. In a discussion of Freud's *Moses and Monotheism,* she says:

> The historical power of the trauma is not just that the experience is repeated after its forgetting, but that it is only in and through its inherent forgetting that it is first experienced at all. And it is this inherent latency of the event that paradoxically explains the peculiar, temporal structure, the belatedness, of the Jews' historical experience.
>
> *(Caruth, 1996, p.17)*

For Herman and Caruth, a lack of verbal narrative is the "wreckage of a story." It is the destruction of consistency and linkage of people, time, space, and affects in memory (Frank, 1995; Adelman, 1995). In this context, the process of recovery consists of weaving the fragments of the traumatic memory into a narrative that constitutes the person's life experience and sense of self. Herman (1992) maintains:

> Out of the fragmented components of frozen imagery and sensation, patient and therapist slowly reassemble an organized, detailed, verbal account … As the narrative closes in on the most unbearable moments, the patient finds it more and more difficult to use words. At times the patient may spontaneously switch to non-verbal methods of communication … Given the "iconic,"

> visual nature of traumatic memories, creating pictures may represent the most effective initial approach to these "indelible images." The completed narrative must include a full and vivid description of the traumatic imagery.
>
> *(Herman, 1992, p.177)*

Here, the analyst's job is still seen as helping his or her patient to follow a plot that makes sense of a rejection of voicing, a denial of spoken sentences, silence, forgetting, or contradictory statements, through movement, gesture, affect, vitality affects, and interactions in analytic dialogue. An analyst works with his or her patient in the belief that the unspoken materials will ultimately come to be articulated and formulated.

The same observation can be made of recent studies in non-narrative in the psychoanalytic process which are *not* necessarily related to trauma. The Boston Change Process Study Group (2007), for example, focuses on human interaction on the "local level" and has organized a pioneering model of non-verbal process that includes movement, gesture, affect, vitality affects, and background feelings—what Daniel Stern (1992) calls the "Pre-Narrative Envelope." This model provides a way of looking at what the unspoken communication means and implies that the analyst's job is to articulate the unspoken processes.

Donnel Stern (2010) innovatively reconceptualizes unconscious life as "unformulated experience" and illustrates the way in which it emerges as an unwitting enactment of the experience in a relational context. While his idea opens up a new way of articulating the therapeutic process from a relational perspective, it does not presuppose the existence of emptiness; there are still two separate but related processes at work: formulated experience and unformulated experience.

In my perspective, these views of narrative in a psychoanalytic process—telling or not-telling, spoken or not-spoken, shattered or not shattered, formulated or not formulated—are all shaped by a Western perspective (I do not deny, however, that it is a cross-cultural predisposition for human beings to view the world as a collection of stories, whether they arise in a distinct narrative form or not). As psychoanalysts we are trained to formulate narratives. An analyst, listening to someone's narrative, attempts to follow a plot; if they are not given a narrative from the other, they try to make sense of, or even create a story about, what is not spoken. If they witness someone's act of narrating, they can tell a story about the act, and if they witness someone's act of not narrating, they can construct a story about non-acting.

A female patient of mine, a professional in her fifties, in three-times a week analysis, struggled to talk about her subjective experiences. She stated that no words or phrases were useful to describe her experiences. If I encouraged her to describe her feelings, she would follow my suggestions, but told me that words wrecked the essence of her subjective feelings. Listening to her description, I found myself automatically searching for narratives that were missed or that I was not aware of. I tried to construct a story about how her subjective experience might not have been organized. It bothered her when I asked her to describe what made it difficult to find appropriate words. She gently told me, "You always try to find a story. I know that it is your job, but I feel the effort doesn't mean anything to me. I just can't talk. There is nothing here." I responded, "I didn't ask you to find a problem in your mind. I think there may be something in our interaction which makes it difficult for you to talk, but I think that together we can find a story that makes sense." She sighed regretfully and said, "What if there is only an empty box?" I had no answer but found myself still thinking that her final statement could be a part of a story of our interaction.

My attitude in this vignette derives from what I call the Western narrative model. I, as a therapist, sought missing stories in two senses. First, I tried to find a story my patient might have not been able to verbalize. Second, I attempted to formulate a narrative to describe how, and in what way, she and I came to reach an impasse organized around non-narrating. I was highly motivated to formulate a narrative; emptiness in my thoughts was intolerable. Even the patient's complaining, "There is nothing," was understood by me as part of the narrative I should—but had not yet be able to—formulate.

Since this episode, I have come to believe that in the fields of relational and narrative psychoanalysis, researchers have not sufficiently called attention to the therapeutic action of emptiness. Eastern perspectives would allow an analyst to accept the possibility that he or she cannot formulate anything from a patient's speech or non-speech. It is not axiomatic that something productive is unfolding in what is spoken or not spoken, or in the action of verbal or non-verbal narrating.

The Eastern idea of emptiness, as I have suggested, does not presuppose a dichotomy of presence and absence. Defining this emptiness is, by definition, a difficult task, especially using traditional Western binary concepts, because Eastern emptiness reflects a nameless and concept-less universe without distinctions between named entities of the world. In the concept-less universe, there is neither presence nor absence.

Emptiness also can be conceptualized as the moment without context, in which neither a sense of being, a living experience, nor a meeting of the other has yet emerged. Spoken is unspoken, and formulated experience is unformulated experience; everything reduced to the moment without context.

I will try to illustrate how a surrender to emptiness can appear in psychoanalytic work, with a vignette of a Japanese female patient who often fell asleep in session, and often remained silent for long periods. While this vignette is intended to explore and develop the concept of surrender through Eastern traditions, I believe that the findings are not culturally specific and can be applied to psychoanalytic work between a Western analyst and Western patient. As Ghent (1990) describes it, surrender can be expressed in many forms, depending on the culture in which it is experienced.

My approach can be seen, in this sense, as contributing to the decolonization of psychoanalysis. Following Hernández-Wolfe, I see a decolonizing perspective "as an alternative departure and as a framework for theory- and practice-building that decenters the status quo of inequities generated and maintained by the cultural, social, and economic capital of dominant groups" (Hernández-Wolfe, 2011, p.294). For psychoanalysts, this is a paradigm shift in which the subject recognizes herself as being embedded within a Western paternalism and attempts to create a new horizon with other perspectives which are not dominated in this way.

Case illustration[1]

Yukiko was a photographer in her early thirties. She entered a four-times a week psychoanalysis on the couch in order to deal with her fear of intimacy. She had few friends, only some professional colleagues, and her social and private lives were separate and isolated.

It was approximately three months after beginning her analysis that I found that Yukiko was falling asleep on the couch. For a few months after, I would wake her up and ask her to explore what might make her do this every session. She did not seem reluctant to accept my requests—she often suggested ideas of her own about her sleeping—but, still, she would end up falling asleep in the midst of talking. All my efforts to keep her engaged and awake would fail, even though, to the best of my knowledge, she had no physical problems that would cause her to fall asleep, nor did she have any medical history of narcolepsy. Indeed, she said that she'd had no previous experience of falling asleep unawares, except for in her sessions with me.

My dilemma was compounded by Yukiko's complaints of a deflation of her creativity. She claimed that she could not reach the essential part of her artistic sensitivity, that whenever she tried to take a photo no feeling or artistic sense came to her mind. She felt that she had almost forgotten how to create a picture with her camera. The more I attempted to explore her falling asleep, the more she complained about the loss of her creativity. I felt helpless and powerless, distressed with her lack of control (and mine) over her sleep and wakefulness.

My understanding at that time was that Yukiko needed to withdraw from the outside world, including me, by shutting down all stimuli. I felt that she was afraid of being intimate with me; that my queries, empathic comments, and interpretations were experienced by her as overwhelming indications of intimacy, and only served to increase her fearful expectations. The story of her relationship with her mother underwrote this perception.

Yukiko's mother, having minor paranoid tendencies, maintained that all people in the world operate with malicious intent. For her, people were untrustworthy, their minds filled with intrigue and conspiracy. She criticized her husband as having a "dirty will," which often made him into a sexual monster. When Yukiko was a little girl, she accepted this perspective. But she came to know that her father was simply not concerned about the human world, dirty or pure, sexual or asexual. He lived in an emotionless world with no space for creativity and the arts. He was deeply self-absorbed and did not seek any meaningful relationship with his family.

My understanding of Yukiko's need to withdraw helped me to create a space in my thoughts. While formerly, I had been desperate to analyze the meaning of Yukiko's sleep and had run through numerous influences and theories, now I no longer pushed. I did not feel that I had to wake her up immediately and discuss her falling asleep. I let her sleep as long as she wanted, typically about thirty minutes. Sitting behind the couch, I spent the time alone with my thoughts and listened to her breathing.

About a year after I stopped pushing to understand it, Yukiko's sleeping in session ended. She also resumed working and actively devoting herself to the photo business. She talked about her way of photographing an object, saying that she always "waited for a moment of nothingness." She began by consciously determining how to shoot the object, and carefully checked any technical issues. Then, she "vanished" her self-consciousness and threw herself into the moment. If she successfully brought herself to this condition, the moment of shooting came to her. "But, now," she said, "I was not able to vanish myself. I waited for the moment with my camera in hand, but 'I' slid into my consciousness. As long as there is a sense of 'I' there, I cannot shoot anything."

Even after she stopped sleeping in session, Yukiko often had periods of silence, frequently for minutes at a time. When I asked her to tell me how she felt during these silences, her reply was ambiguous; "I don't know. My mind was just empty." If I had not experienced a year of her sleep sessions, I would have aggressively analyzed this state. I tried not to explore it as actively as I might have done, and I allowed her to make time for silence. I tried to stay with her, keeping my arousal and physiological state at a low level. As long as I kept myself in this state, she also stayed calm and felt easy. Toward the end of the third year of her analysis, she said to me, "Silence is silence. If you want, it is okay to talk about this, but I think that it is a waste of time. Don't focus on the silence."

One day Yukiko told me about a dream in which she found herself in a snow-covered town where there were no other human beings. Houses, trees, roads, and all other objects were blanketed with snow as far as the eye could see. In the dream, she was excited at the prospect of taking photos of the scene because she could see "the real faces" of all objects.

I wondered if, through this dream, Yukiko was struggling to capture the essence of the world, the essence of her aesthetic. She needed a space which was not contaminated by her mother's paranoid filter. For her, language, exploration, and interpretation were not pure white like the snow-covered world she saw in the dream; they were all potentially contaminated by her basic mistrust of the world. As long as she was asleep or in silence, she could feel secure enough to capture this essence of the world. In other words, she attempted to move through nothingness toward essence. I finally recognized that my efforts at interpretation and narrative exploration were not helping and may have been meaningless. There was no story to be found. I had to stop "thinking" and let go of my search for an immediate explanation.

For the last year of her analysis, Yukiko no longer fell asleep or maintained notable silences in session, and I found that a unique rhythm had emerged between us, organized around a matched pause. As she finished talking, almost simultaneously I stopped thinking, and my mind became empty for a short time. This is unusual for me. Typically, as I listen to my patients I sense that my brain is working actively and processing all the information I obtain from their narrations and behaviors. Toward the end of their speaking, my brain activity rises to a climax, and then, immediately after they finish, I give them my thoughts and feelings. But in the relationship with Yukiko, we both achieved an empty moment simultaneously; I found myself not thinking anything. If I had not experienced her sleeping and silence for the first three years of analysis, I could not have recognized and accepted this phenomenon.

In one session, Yukiko talked about a short trip she had made with a male colleague at a web company's request. She was nervous and felt uncomfortable being with him for the whole day. As she began to talk, I found my brain working very hard. What was it she wanted to say through this episode? Was she expressing the essential conflict? What did she expect me to say? As usual, I constructed a story in my mind for each issue and attempted to articulate the highest priority at each moment: intimacy with others, trust for others, or a yearning to share some feeling with me. In this case, however, as Yukiko finished her story, my thoughts slowed down and came to a stop. There was a pause. The pause was a very short, but our communication and my internal activities were both suspended; probably her level of internal activity went down, too.

After this, Yukiko began to feel more comfortable and more like herself when being with others. She developed a good reputation in her field and no longer feared that her creativity was being contaminated by the thoughts of others. She said, "the sense of art in my soul is uniquely my own, but it helps me to connect to the world and others. The sense of art is everywhere." She terminated analysis after four years when she was offered a good position with a large company in another city.

Discussion and conclusion—narrative as the zero

Working with Yukiko showed how deeply I, as her analyst, was focused on formulating a narrative. When I faced her sleeping and silence, I automatically searched for meaning by attempting to create a story, to construct a narrative that could explain how sleeping and silence came to be organized in the therapeutic process. When I constructed this kind of story, I referred to plot points in her childhood, her professional work, her dreams, and in our therapeutic interactions. I pieced the information together so as to make it spatially structured and temporally consistent. But all my efforts only seemed to further her anguish.

By contrast, what would it have meant to surrender myself to Yukiko's *emptiness*? It would have meant not constructing a story and freeing myself from my preoccupation with formulating a narrative. The process I am describing is not about finding a non-narrated story, or finding a meaning in Yukiko's non-narrating; it is about relinquishing the narrative altogether. This stance of surrender helped me find a way of working with and relating to Yukiko. Of course, I also recognize the irony that in sharing this case in a coherent fashion, I have, in a sense, imposed a narrative framework on my work with Yukiko. The narrative process of case formulation is nevertheless taking place in hindsight and, as such, is different from the moments of "emptiness" that I have described in my work with my patient.

In Western psychoanalysis, we are trained to find what it is that transpires during an interaction. Even when we encounter a silence or pause, we seek to understand what meaning it might have. But as Yukiko's case suggests, a psychological process can often be organized around the moment of emptiness. A Bionian analyst, Boris (1986, 1987) maintains the importance of tolerating a notion of "nothing" in psychoanalytic process, pointing out that for many analysts, including Bion, "there is no such thing as nothing" (Boris, 1987, p.351). In response, Boris criticizes the traditional analyst's necessity for seeking meaning or the presence of absence in silence or no-actions. He says:

> One's own capacity to tolerate nothing quickly becomes an issue central to the analysis. If one can regard the torment of experience as a hateful fact, analysis is possible. If one succumbs to the temptation to replace the no-things with something—well one soon is out of the analysis business and into the transfusion business.
>
> *(Boris, 1987, p.365)*

Boris's (1987) notion is innovative and helpful, but his emphasis is still on an analyst's ability to accept "absence" or "nothingness" rather than emptiness. Emptiness means neither absence nor nothingness. It is beyond the distinction between presence and absence. It is nothing and everything and is the essence of the world. We can see a good example in Yukiko's case. Her original silence was not emptiness, but nothingness, a silence organized in a context in which she left herself free from non-recognition by her father and the malignant paranoia of her mother. That was her "pathological accommodation" (Brandchaft, Doctors, & Sorter, 2010) to that perspective. But Yukiko's and my letting go of "our" search for a story and an immediate explanation about her silence was, instead, a moment without context. If it had been our effort to accommodate to her silence, she would have needed to protect herself from my preoccupation with searching for a story.

How can we describe the intersubjective field in which Yukiko accessed the essence of the world or the essence of her aesthetic? I believe what dissolved the analytic impasse in Yukiko's case was our surrender to the "moment of nothingness," as she called it. For her, words and memories were contaminated by other people's perspectives, mostly her mother's. The essence of a human relationship, for her, could only be created through a process in which we both renounced the necessity to formulate narratives. Yukiko, an artist, seemed to know how to create an essential moment. She also knew how the moment had the potential to create a secure and *trust-able* world. In other words, the moment included the essence of the world and human relationships. By relinquishing our attempts to think, explore, analyze, and focus on her psychological condition, Yukiko and I surrendered ourselves to a relational system which moved to a calm stillness, emptiness. I refer to this process as the *psychoanalytic zero*, the concept that I (Togashi, 2016b, 2017c, 2017d, 2017e, 2017g) maintained, in a series of phenomenological studies of an Asian sense of responsibility and ethics, as a new perspective of the ethical turn in psychoanalysis.

In this chapter, I have attempted to expand Ghent's (1990) idea of surrender, especially in relation to emptiness. Surrender can be to emptiness, the moment without context, in which neither a sense of being, a living experience, nor a meeting with the other has yet emerged. Surrendering to emptiness allows an analyst to go beyond spoken and unspoken narratives, formulated or unformulated experiences, or named or unnamed phenomena to be sensitive to the essence of the world, Nature.

Surrendering to emptiness is the essential aspect of the psychoanalytic zero. For me, emptiness does not refer to a special moment, but can be found anywhere in the psychoanalytic process. It can be felt anywhere we allow ourselves to accept the essence of the world, the *Taoist Nature*. In a spontaneous conversation a narrator does not deliver a fully constructed and plotted narrative and, moment by moment, does not know exactly what he or she will say or how it will be understood by the other. A narrator does not know which element in the ocean of memory will surface in the next moment and become part of the story. In a dialogue, no one can predict where a narrative will go; the narrator can only let go of his or herself and take in the moment as it is. If a narrator or a listener attempts to process all the available information, he or she must fail to capture the essence of the dialogue or the relationship, because they limit the infinite possibilities of the moment.

In this sense, emptiness does not only appear in sleep, silence, or pause; it can also occur in our normal dialogue. In Yukiko's case, the moment of nothingness was the center of the therapeutic action. In this state, she could transcend the guilt of being (Togashi, 2017c, and see also Chapter 2), which came from her fears of contaminating me with her basic mistrust about the world and being contaminated by my personal view of the world. All mental activities and intersubjective processes were stilled, yet within this state lay a great potential for creating the essence of our relationship: trust, a sense of security, the sense of selves, subjectivity, our interactions, and her creativity.

Emptiness, the psychoanalytic zero, emerges prior to an analyst's and a patient's awareness of their identities, their sense of self, and their professional, therapeutic, social, and cultural roles. Emptiness may or may not be embodied in a silent space, but it does not have a temporal consistency or spatial structure in itself. It may reside at the center of anything in the analytic relationship; it does not have anything, yet it can create anything.

Note

1 This clinical case is discussed in greater detail in Chapter 4.

2

BEYOND THE GUILT OF BEING

Surrender to emptiness

A male Japanese patient claims, "I should not have been born in this world because I am nothing." A female patient repeatedly says, "Everyone will be happy if I die. I don't deserve to live in this world. But I cannot kill myself because that will cause trouble for someone."

Practicing psychoanalysis in the Far East, it is not unusual for me to see patients like these. Although they inflict no harm on other people, have no dangerous thoughts or ideations, do not violate the basic rules of the human world or engage in prohibited conduct, they nonetheless feel that they are worthless sinners and that their existence makes other people feel bad. Although these patients are quite sensitive to how other people feel about them, they do not develop severe paranoid symptoms. This condition has been seen in Japanese psychiatry and psychoanalysis as a culture-bound syndrome of neurasthenia or anthropophobia (Uchinuma, 1977, 1981, 1983; Morita, 1921; Okano, 1994, 1998).

These patients suffer feelings of ethical responsibility for transgressions they have committed prior to encountering the other; transgressions that have nothing to do with their intentions, behaviors, wishes or actions, but with their very being in this world. In their minds, from the moment of their birth, or even before, they have been designated as scum who generate nothing but harmful effects for people and society.

The ethical responsibility these patients feel does not completely fit among Freudian ethical transgressions. These patients do not experience incestuous wishes or fantasies, nor do they feel responsible for behaviors corresponding to any level of intentionality—unintended accidents, carelessness, deliberate recklessness, or fully intentional and purposeful acts (Meissner, 2003; Gutkin, 1973). Neither is their guilt relevant to care ethics. These patients do not feel ashamed of not being able to respond to the call for help from the other. Nor do they feel ashamed of their being in a safe place when other people are in danger. Rather, they believe that their misconduct was committed before encountering the other, or even before being born. Their experience may be characterized as, "I apologize for having made you feel bad before I showed up on your doorstep. If I had not been in this world, I would not have made you feel awful."

The ethical responsibility these patients experience may be rooted in East Asian culture, which tends to see the world as an inherently open system in which the karmic chain is included in itself. Many East Asian philosophical schools, including Buddhism, Confucianism, and *Taoism*, find the origin of their ethics in the notion of an infinite universe.

These patients anguish over not being able to find a way to compensate for their transgressions. Such compensation is not so easily found in our clinical practice, of course, because their sins are neither acts, intentions, fantasies, harms, injuries, damage to others, or incompetent caregiving skills. Their crime is simply being in this world, and they feel that the ultimate form of atonement they could make would be to delete themselves. But they believe that their transgressions can never be erased completely, even after their death, and there is nothing they can do to atone for their sins.

One patient, Hitomi, a professional Japanese female in her thirties, believed that her presence made other people feel bad. She never doubted in the slightest that she did not deserve to live in this world. She assumed a cheerful demeanor in her office, but secretly worried that she was detested by her colleagues. In my office, she always looked down and avoided making eye contact with me.

Hitomi was unable to have intimate relationships with others regardless of gender. I suggested to her that fear of intimacy might be caused by a fear of being touched by emotional experiences. Her response, delivered in her typically apologetic manner, was "It isn't like that. I am annoying, that's it." I did not understand what she meant at the time and felt that her answer only confirmed the rightness of my understanding. But I came to see that this was a mistake on my part.

Several months later, I commented on a unique behavior of Hitomi's. I usually open the door to invite my patients into my office so that they pass by me as they enter. I found that Hitomi habitually walked with her head down and never looked at my face when she entered. When I told her that I was concerned about this behavior, she said, "You don't understand how terrible I feel about coming to this office" She looked down and continued, "I don't deserve to sit here, not because I am afraid of being touched with my emotions, but because I make *you* feel bad. I don't have a problem feeling my emotional experience; the problem is that I am *me*." She was convinced that I was bothered by her being, and she felt guilty about taking up my time and energy. She fully believed that she should give up her regular session to someone more worthy of my time. Yet, she also believed that the patient who could take over her time could not be happy because the appointment time would always be tainted by its association with her, a hopeless sinner.

What can psychoanalysts do when they see a patient like Hitomi? Interpretation and comment, attempts to reassure or be with the patient and mirror her being—none of this could help. Rather, these efforts would be bound to make her feel worse, because she would feel that she was forcing her therapist to concentrate on her as well as know that he or she would not have needed to make such efforts if they did not see her.

I believe that what therapists can do for a patient like Hitomi is not to do anything while being with them. The patient's self-perceived transgression is that their very being hurts others, and therapists' efforts to treat, reassure, and change them only compound this sin. The only ways in which the patient would not feel transgressive in this intersubjective field would be to free herself and her therapist from any preoccupation with good or bad, doable or undoable, and right or wrong.

In this chapter, I propose an Asian perspective on the "*ethical turn*" in psychoanalysis. I explore a psychoanalytic understanding of the anguish of patients who feel guilt about their being and illustrate a process of working through it. I argue that, to transcend the guilt of being, therapists and patients are required to surrender themselves to *emptiness*, in which both participants efface the preoccupation with themselves in the presence of each other, leaving a field beyond right and wrong, or good and bad.

Guilt of being

Patients who feel guilty for simply *existing* believe that they cause trouble to others simply by being in this world, and also by not being. In Japan, this type of patient has been well-known for a long time. They often enact their guilt or shame in symptoms such as Morita neurosis (culturally-bound constitutional neurasthenia), and culturally-bound anthropophobia including four subtypes: the fear of blushing (*sekimen-kyofu*), fear of a deformed body (*shubo-kyofu*), fear of one's own glance (*jikoshisen-kyofu*), and the fear of one's own foul body odor (*jikoshu-kyofu*) (Hofmann, Asnaani, & Hinton, 2010).

Uchinuma (1977, 1981, 1983) suggests that this anthropophobia is a culturally unique expression of interpersonal conflicts such as "self-centeredness vs. other-centeredness," "selfishness vs. selflessness," and "separation vs. merger." A unique contribution of his theory is understanding the treatment process to be one of ethical development, in which a feeling of shame is transformed to a feeling of embarrassment, then guilt, and finally to a state beyond right and wrong. In this discussion, shame and guilt are experientially close and located in one developmental line. He suggests that a therapeutic moment is often built in a non-conflict space between the two extremes of the interpersonal situation; the space which patients surrender themselves to by releasing a preoccupation with self, other, and society. I believe this space can be seen as emptiness, or what *Taoism* calls Nature, from which everything is born and to which everything is reduced.

The Morita therapy, which is a culturally unique therapeutic intervention for a similar type of patient, includes the idea of a non-conflict space in its therapeutic process. The original form of this therapy, developed in the 1920s by a Japanese psychiatrist, Morita, consists of four stages—isolation and rest, light occupational work, intensive occupational work, and preparation for daily living—which are usually given in a residential treatment facility. The therapeutic goal is to arrive at a pure state of mind in which patients are freed from a "fixation" with their unsuccessful attempts to cope with their inner conflicts. The key to this process is that patients are expected to commit to a state in which they efface or suspend all concern about themselves, others, and their environment.

The ethical dimension in these models is different from that in usual Western psychoanalytic models, in which the moral imperative for patients is understood to be an integrative self that allows them to take responsibility for deliberation, choice, and action (Meissner, 2003). In these traditional Japanese models, on the other hand, the moral ideal for patients is considered to be attaining the state of selflessness and *otherlessness*. It is not until patients relinquish their preoccupation with themselves, others, their environment, and society that they can achieve a state beyond good and bad, or right and wrong. It is no wonder that these treatment models do not include a process for working through transference, for dealing with transference means that patients are expected to focus on themselves and others.

The psychoanalysts who work with these guilt-ridden patients have to be ready to abandon their own preoccupations with themselves, their patients, and their professional environment –in essence, effacing their professional identities to surrender themselves to *emptiness* in the intersubjective field before their patients can be free from the guilt of being. In this perspective, which I call *the psychoanalytic zero*, therapist and patient can say to each other, "I want you to know that I am here, too; but remember, I am also not here."

A moment without distinction between presence and absence

The concept of *emptiness,* or zero, has not been sufficiently discussed in the psychoanalytic field. What psychoanalytic researchers and clinicians have mostly elaborated is "nothingness" or "absence" rather than emptiness. Freud indicated his interest in "no" or "negative" in his book, *Interpretation of Dreams* (1900–01). He emphasized that there is no "no" in the unconscious and argued that dreams have no way to manifest content that expresses a negative. For Freud, any "no" or "negative" is either the approximation of a repression or a denial of something unacceptable. In other words, in his model, there is no notion of nothingness; absence refers to a state in which something is missed or rejected.

Freud (1920a, 1924) later addressed the question of how psychic processes are controlled in a living organism. For him, this organic system is the *nirvana principle*, "the effort to reduce, to keep constant or to remove internal tension due to stimuli" (Freud, 1920a, 55–56). Freud's position, however, is quite ambiguous. At one point (1920a, 1924), he maintains that the nirvana principle belongs to the death instinct "whose aim is to conduct the restlessness of life into the stability of the inorganic state, and it [the nirvana principle] would have the function of giving warnings against the demands of the life instincts" (Freud, 1924, p.160). But in other writings he assigns it to the "pleasure principle" (Freud, 1924, p.159), the tendency to reduce all tension to a point of nothing. Freud never refers to a point of nothing as absence of tension, but always as a reference point in a principle of constancy.

For post-Freudian analysts, there is no significant difference in this basic understanding of nothing. Most traditional ego psychologists see silence and wordlessness in patients as resistance or a dissociated mental state. For these analysts, the phenomena are subjects for interpretation or exploration in order to illustrate the hidden stories behind them (Greenson, 1967; Arlow, 1961). More recent theorists, such as Ronningstam (2006), do not immediately see the patient's failure to verbalize something as resistance or an effort to hide something from the analyst. They recognize the cultural meaning of nothing and value it in the therapeutic or developmental process. Yet, in their understandings, nothing still indicates *something*, such as a relational pattern or complicated developmental process.

Contemporary psychoanalytic narrative theories and relational theorists see *nothing* in the same vein, as discussed in Chapter 1. They conceptualize what is unspoken as an expression of something that has been disavowed, unformulated, or remains unorganized or not allowed to be told, and there are always some such stories for the patient and analyst to find.

I want to emphasize here that the problem in these discussions is not that they do not accept a notion of absence or nothing, but that they retain the distinction between some-thing and no-thing, or presence and absence, in the human mind, human relationships, and society. In these theories, all entities are defined as either present or absent.

One psychoanalytic thinker who does go beyond the distinction between presence and absence is Wilfred Bion. In his elaboration of different kinds of knowing, he proposes the notion of K, knowing and cognizing, and O, a state of unknowing, which is the ground of being, an ultimate unknowable reality or formless infinite.

> I shall use the sign O to denote that which is the ultimate reality represented by terms such as ultimate reality, absolute truth, the godhead, the infinite, the thing-in-itself. O does not fall in the domain of knowledge or learning save incidentally; it can be "become," but it cannot be "known." It is darkness and formlessness, but it enters the domain K when it has evolved to a point where it can be known, through knowledge gained by experience, and formulated in terms derived from sensuous experience; its existence is conjectured phenomenologically.
>
> (Bion, 1970, p. 26)

This statement suggests that K means the evolution of O. O does not refer to not-knowing or the absence of knowing, but to seeing things in themselves in therapists' efforts to embrace emptiness. As Mendoza (2010) argues in his creative writings, Bion's concept is seen as similar to the Buddhist notion of emptiness, which is not absence or vacuum, but leads to wisdom. Like Buddhist emptiness, the notion of O employs the dual view in which two different experiences go hand in hand, such as thinking and feeling, form and content, and container and contained. The inherent existence of phenomena and their fullness of experience and aesthetics emerge in the moment in which the two different experiences find themselves in each other; to be content is to be form, and to be contained is to be a container.

Bion (1970) suggests that the analyst be unknown so that he or she may be filled by their patient. He states:

> The analyst must focus his attention on O, the unknown and unknowable. The success of psycho-analysis depends on the maintenance of a psycho-analytic point of view; the point of view is the psycho-analytic vertex; the psychoanalytic vertex is O. With this the analyst cannot be identified: he must *be* it.
>
> *(Bion, 1970, p.27; emphasis in original)*

For Bion (1970), the analyst's job is not to know about his or her patient, but to become the O, the essence and true nature of his or her patient.

My concept of the psychoanalytic zero is very close to Bion's notion of O, but there are still a few differences (despite the curious similarity between the two symbols, 0 for zero and O). Unlike O, the zero does not refer to the ground of being or ultimate nature of the patient, but to an aspect of Nature emerging in the infinite universe or in analytic work. In other words, the zero is neither something in the patient, nor the analyst, nor in the relationship between them. I do not suggest that the analyst must *be* zero, but that he or she is required to surrender him or herself to emptiness. Another point of departure from Bion is that the psychoanalytic zero model does not entail *knowing* in its evolution. The psychoanalytic zero may or may not be connected to the analyst's knowing, but instead requires an intersubjective process in which two people efface their preoccupation with themselves by surrendering to the moment without context, the primal moment of human encounter in our clinical practice.

Case vignette

Hitomi, the patient I described earlier, came to see me complaining of depression and minor depersonalization. She was occasionally preoccupied with a suicidal fantasy in which she hanged herself from the ceiling. She was an intelligent professional with a good reputation in her field, but she felt she had no reason for living. She was afraid of being physically close to others, regardless of gender, and believed that her existence made other people feel bad. When she felt that way, she saw no alternative other than killing herself.

I had seen her for four years on a twice-a-week basis, face to face. For the first year of her therapy, I was confused by her repetitive expression of a wish to kill herself. She said, "I am a terrible person and a worthless sinner. I want to disappear, but I do not want to kill myself because that would only cause you trouble. I cannot go anywhere. But I should delete myself." She strongly believed that her presence was a terrible burden to me. Although I reassured her that there was no reason to see herself as a sinner, and that I did not at all feel bothered by her, she clung to her belief in her own worthlessness. Occasionally, I could tell that my attempts to make her feel better actually made her feel worse. I felt powerless and helpless, which seemed to reinforce her feeling that her presence was a hardship to me, even though I did not voice my frustration in session. She often said that she needed to leave therapy although she wanted to keep coming. This stalemate continued for several months until I reached some understanding about the sources of her anguish, sparked by our discussion about her not looking at my face, as described above.

After nearly a year and a half, Hitomi related a fantasy that effaced both of us, but which allowed her to feel more comfortable about coming to my office. She said, "I know that this is crazy, but I feel that you are in the moon and I am on the earth but I am invisible." When I asked her to describe her fantasy further, she said, "I am not sure where I am, but I can see the moon, where you live. I cannot figure out you, though." I had no idea what this fantasy meant and did not get a clear explanation about it from her. There was no understanding we could share about the meaning of this fantasy. Hitomi emphasized, however, that she felt it easier to be in my office as long as she could picture our relationship in this way.

At this point, we were able to talk about her background. Hitomi was the only daughter of an unsophisticated working-class couple. They did not understand the intellectual curiosity that she developed in her early years, and they often made it clear that they despised her. Her mother, who had a minor paranoid tendency, told her that they had not wanted a child, and that Hitomi had no need of an education, except to learn nursing-care techniques, claiming that the only reason they'd had Hitomi was to take care of them when they became older. The mother denigrated her daughter's interests in literature. Hitomi's mother had passed away several years before she came to see me, but the father was still alive, although alcoholic and frequently hospitalized. He littered their home with broken, cast-off appliances that he would collect but never attempt to repair. After his wife died, he was dependent on Hitomi economically and psychologically, and required her to take care of him.

This history made it easier to understand why Hitomi felt herself to be a meaningless and worthless sinner. I was no longer surprised by her assertion that she did not deserve to live and take up my time. For her, the only reason she was alive was to take care of her father. She believed that, as her mother had insisted, her intellectual curiosity was silly and worthless. On one occasion, I interpreted her belief as being linked to her relationship with her parents, and on another, reassured her that I, unlike her parents, did not feel bothered by her intellectual interests, but Hitomi said that she already knew my understandings and she could not accept my reassurances. Rather, she felt apologetic for making me spend my energy and time trying to understand her and give comments. I felt disappointed in myself. Nothing I could do was effective, and the harder I worked to understand her, the guiltier she felt.

When Hitomi told me her moon story, I thought it was interesting and beautiful, and I was attracted by her intelligent worldview. She had a good sense of literary aesthetics, and the fantasies and stories she described for me easily held my attention. When I told her honestly that I enjoyed her story, she went pale and shamefully said, "I am so sorry. Forget about everything."

I was surprised and said, "Tell me why you want me to forget about the story."

"Because the story is worthless and I feel sorry for your spending your energy to listen to it."

"Why? I really like the story."

"If so, all the worse. You spent your important time and energy to understand this story. I know I need you, which is why I am here in therapy. But I don't feel I deserve to be your patient. I don't like to bother you."

"I am confused. I told you that I enjoyed the story, which means that I was happy to hear it. What makes you feel you don't deserve to be my patient? It sounds like you do not want *me* to feel happy."

"No. I want you to be happy. Therefore you should not see me. You are too much present to me. When I become aware of you here in the room, I feel awful."

I finally understood that my presence strongly affected her. My being seemed to be harmful to her, and no matter what I said, even positive remarks, would have some influence over her. I asked myself if I had ever seriously considered how much my voice, tone, gaze, language, and actions stirred her emotions. The answer was no. I was aware that both a so-called neutral or analytic abstinence attitude, and an "anything-goes" attitude could be harmful, but I was not aware of the fact that, for this patient, *any* action on the part of the therapist could be harmful, in the sense that the patient had to deal with the influence she was exposed to. Even given a positive affirmation, she would be forced to consider whether or not she could trust my words; whether there were any hidden messages in my words; whether she had experienced similar affirmations before in her life, and why or why not; and whether she was really good, etc.

In psychoanalytic psychotherapy, the patient continually sees her therapist waiting for her response. She is granted significant freedom to respond in her own way, but she immediately knows that her mind is already eroded by her own history and by her therapist's expectations. She anguishes over being at liberty to say anything to someone who is in her presence for a purpose.

The original moon fantasy in which both Hitomi and I were invisible implied that she had to avoid finding me and she should disappear from my presence, even though she wanted to be with me. I had to be invisible; otherwise, my very being stimulated her feelings and made her feel terrible. I recognized that I had to abandon my own preoccupation, my wish to be a good therapist (to cure Hitomi, take care of her, enjoy her stories and provide insightful comments, etc), even my own preoccupation with understanding her. It was necessary that whatever Hitomi said, I simply listened and talked about it without interpreting the content of the story or the way she brought it into the therapeutic field.

A few sessions later, we returned to Hitomi's original story of the moon. As usual, she maintained that she did not appear anywhere in this story. I made no reply, which was unusual, but remained silent. She glanced at me, awaiting my comments. I simply said, "It is interesting. Maybe I am on the moon, but I could not say where precisely."

"You are there, though."

"Yes. But a human figure would be invisible. What we can see is only the moon."

"What do you mean by that?"

"I don't know. I just said something that popped into my mind, that's all. No interpretation here."

She smiled and went on to another topic.

The significant aspect of this exchange was what took place in the unvoiced area. I had stopped reflecting on our therapeutic work in a psychoanalytic way. I showed no evidence of making any effort on her behalf, and Hitomi probably had no idea what was in my mind. Abandoning a preoccupation with my role as a therapist, I sought no understanding, no association, and no interpretation. I was just there. This change, however, created a unique rhythm between us. *No-thinking* states, which often manifested in occasional silences and even in conversation, emerged in our intersubjective field. In such a state we worked together with no orientation, no expectation, and no purpose. We did not know which way our talk would go, but simply let it go where it would.

Towards the end of her therapy, Hitomi was no longer afraid of looking at me. She now brought her gaze to my face. Her basic humility had not changed very much, but she did not feel herself as a terrible sinner anymore. Further, she became energetic and more cheerful. For the last year of her therapy, our sessions remained like this. We did a lot of talking, all without plans, aims, or predetermined goals. We surrendered ourselves to a process with no pre-determined professional name, abandoning all self-preoccupations about our therapeutic work. It was not always easy for us to hold onto this state, because those self-preoccupations were always ready to slide into our minds. But as long as we stayed in it, Hitomi could allow herself to live in this world.

Four years after we began working together, Hitomi made a decision to enroll in graduate school in a new field. She no longer felt herself as a burden, even though she felt an urge to take care of me. She said, "I would do anything for you if you need my help. I am no longer afraid of myself. I believe that if I had said this before, I would have felt myself being harmful to you." I simply said, "Thank you. Your concern is accepted."

Conclusion and discussion

Hitomi was overwhelmed by a sense of guilt over her own existence, the simple fact of her being. She believed that her presence made me feel bad, and my attempts to show support or concern did not help because she could not accept that she might deserve my consideration. She felt, rather, that she must apologize for being a burden to me. When she experienced herself as sinful, she fantasized about deleting herself, often in the form of suicidal ideation.

Hitomi's felt guilt was neither a response to inhibited unconscious wishes, nor to fantasies in which she hurt me, but for a transgression committed prior to encountering me. This transgression did not have to do with her intentions, behaviors, wishes, or actions; but with her very being in this world. As her therapist, my psychoanalytic interventions dealing with transference issues made her feel worse, because such an effort, by her therapist, became the very transgression she felt she had to take responsibility for.

The therapeutic moment that broke this stalemate was my surrendering myself to the *emptiness*, in which I abandoned a self-centered concern with my role as a therapist. I proceeded to talk with Hitomi with no clear plans, aims, or destinations, and this change created a unique rhythm in our dialogue, including silent moments, as Hitomi and I allowed ourselves to go with this flow. Abandoning our preoccupations with ourselves created the moment in which we both experienced ourselves as free. This is what I call the *zero*, a moment in which we could be free from right and wrong, good and bad.

Surrendering to emptiness is not an easy job for people, especially therapists. Therapists are trained to perceive and interpret their patients' narratives with a certain purpose and intention. But, as seen in the case vignette, they have to be aware that their personal, social, and professional roles can often make their patients feel terrible.

How can therapists surrender themselves to emptiness? In Hitomi's case, what made surrender possible for me was my recognition of my own transgression. I became aware that I was an overwhelming presence for her, and no matter what I thought and felt, or how I behaved, my being had a considerable impact on her, either positively or negatively. My sin was my being in the same world with her. Without this recognition, I could neither have abandoned all my preoccupations nor allowed myself to be fully present with Hitomi.

We psychoanalysts are guilty of inexpiable offenses. From the moment we show up in the presence of our patients, and even before, we stir their emotions. We inquire into the meaning of their being, we provide kindness that our patients may not be able to compensate for. Still we have to be with our patients. We are in their presence and cannot get away from them whether or not we understand them, whether or not our comments disturb them, whether or not our appearance may make them feel uncomfortable. I would say that this is our sin as therapists.

In my understanding, the sin comes from showing up as a human being. If we were not human beings, our patients would not feel themselves guilty. Because we are human beings, our patients are stimulated by all of our actions and words. Because we are human beings, we are often self-preoccupied; wishing to be skillful therapists and providing too much love and kindness for our patients. We get involved in our patients' worlds as they are involved in ours. When we understand how it is that a sinful, human therapist and a sinful, human patient encounter one another in a small office and attempt to take responsibility for the lives and the sins they have not chosen, we can surrender ourselves to emptiness.

3

AN ASIAN ETHICAL PERSPECTIVE ON SINCERITY IN PSYCHOANALYSIS

Psychoanalysts treat their patients within a professional setting. Traditional psychoanalytic models, which emphasize professional and social roles, maintain that the essential feature of the psychoanalyst's job is to employ a technical method for removing or curing a patient's mental problems. In these models, the analyst's commitment to their patient consists of these professional instructions and understandings.

Contemporary psychoanalytic thinkers, however, suggest that the practice of psychoanalysis is not necessarily limited to the professional mindset. They recognize that analysts' personal feelings and thoughts constitute core elements of psychoanalytic work, and often play a significant role in therapeutic interactions. The analyst's human responsibility and compassion for their patients becomes the basis of a human relationship between them, and provides a human experience to the patient.

The effort to bridge the gap between professional and personal responses has been much discussed as part of two developing trends in psychoanalysis: the *relational* and *ethical* trends. While personal and subjective feelings may be congruent with one's professional utterances, it often happens that there is an oppositional tension between them. The relational movement in psychoanalysis pays attention to the ways in which analysts and patients sublate this tension in a therapeutic field (Benjamin, 1990, 1995; Mitchell, 1993, 1997, 2000; Aron, 1996; Hoffman, 1998). These authors associate the analyst's *professional* attitude with neutrality, abstinence, blank screen, and ritual; while self-disclosure, openness, authenticity, and spontaneity are seen as corresponding to an attitude that allows analysts to bring their personal and subjective feelings into the therapeutic field. These authors stress that it is important for the analyst and patient to create a *potential* space, in which they can take both professional *and* personal roles.

While the relational turn places an emphasis on sublating tensions that emerge *after* a patient and an analyst are aware of their professional and personal beings, the *ethical turn* in psychoanalysis (Baraitser, 2008; Corpt, 2013; Brothers, 2014; Orange, 2013, 2014a, 2015; Sucharov, 2014; Weisel-Barth, 2015; Togashi, 2017a) raises the question of how analysts encounter patients *prior to* this awareness, and asks analysts to pay attention to the ways in which they and their patients encounter each other as human beings. For example, Baraitser (2008) criticizes Benjamin's (1995) theory of mutual recognition by saying that it puts too much emphasis on a mother's subjectivity. She proposes that the basis of human ethics is a caregiver responding to the call for responsibility from her baby, the Other, even before being aware of herself or her role as mother. She describes the Levinasian ethics that provide the theoretical basis for her argument as follows:

> Levinas's argument is in a different register from that of sameness and difference, recognition and reciprocity. Recognition, as discussed earlier, is not identical with responsibility. Self-recognition that relies on recognition by another subject will perhaps always run into difficulties with how to prevent a collapse of alterity due to the colonizing impulse that is inherent not only in "knowing" another but in recognizing too. In contrast, describing the relationship with the Other as an ethical relationship prior to self, a relationship that establishes the subject as a responsible subject before being a subject at all, Levinas redefines both the notion of the subject and the Other as well as the nature of their relationship and that of recognition itself.
>
> *(Baraitser, 2008, p. 102)*

This statement indicates that a caregiver's human responsibility precedes a social or professional role, the awareness of how her self has been established, and does not contradict it in the ethical field. The radical ethics of human responsibility are always already there at the very moment of human encounter, even in a professional encounter. If a patient came into the office bleeding after being injured in a car accident in the street outside, we would immediately take care of him or her, and not be too concerned with maintaining an analytical face.

This perspective makes it clear that there is, ultimately, no dichotomy between our humanity and professionalism. Still, in our clinical encounter with our patients, our human responsibility often comes into question. Is my response to my patient human enough? Is my sincere care for my patient sufficiently professional? Analysts are often confused about how to balance their spontaneous, often personal, human responsibilities with professional appropriateness.

I focus, in this chapter, on "sincerity" in psychoanalytic work, from a decolonizing perspective and within the ethical trend. In my understanding, issues of sincerity appear where our professional responsibility and personal devotion to our patients intersect. When we find ourselves being overly professional, we ask ourselves if we are being sincere as human beings; when we experience ourselves as being too personal, we ask if we have been sincere with our patients as professional therapists. Sincerity is, indeed, one of the most significant concepts in ethics. In the psychoanalytic literature, however, there are only a few articles discussing sincerity directly.

Many contemporary analysts (Mitchell, 1997; Levenson, 1996; Renik, 1995, 1998, 1999; Hoffman, 1998; Teicholz, 2000; Van der Heide, 2007; Benjamin, 2010) have discussed ideas related to sincerity, including honesty, authenticity, autonomy, self-disclosure, integrity, and enactment. These practitioners recognize that it often becomes an important therapeutic action for analysts to disclose their personal feelings and thoughts openly and honestly. Despite some differences of emphasis, they all argue that an analyst's authenticity and spontaneity are basic premises of a therapeutic relationship. Their discussions are innovative in the sense that they challenge the traditional psychoanalytic model, which requires analysts to conceal their personal and honest feelings behind a professional role.

Sincerity is, however, not quite the same as honesty and openness. Sincerity does not necessarily refer to the state of one's mind or behavior. It is an ethical and aesthetic quality in how a person sees and relates to the Other. One can never be certain of his or her true feelings, cannot fully open oneself or present perfect authenticity. Yet, one can be sincere in a relationship with the other while accepting his or her inability to achieve this perfect honesty and openness. One is not always injured by the other's not being open or telling the whole truth; but one can be injured by the other's insincerity.

What is sincerity in psychoanalytic work? How does sincerity function in a psychoanalytic field? In this chapter, I will compare a Western concept of sincerity, as posited in some psychoanalytic articles, with a Japanese ethical concept of sincerity called *makoto,* or *sheijitsu,* and explore the meaning of *makoto*/sincerity as it manifests itself in a living moment of human encounter in psychoanalytic practice.

I begin by reviewing the psychoanalytic discussion on *sincerity* and related concepts, and then compare that with *makoto*/sincerity in Japan. Through a clinical vignette of a female patient with keloid scars on her face, I will illustrate how we might apply *makoto* in psychoanalytic practice. Finally, I will suggest the ways in which *makoto* unfolds in the intersubjective field *before* analysts are aware of their professional and personal considerations.

Sincerity in psychoanalysis

Walker (1978), a British philosopher, identifies two aspects of sincerity. The first is sincerity as truthfulness: truth-telling and ensuring that one's utterance and actions are congruent with one's mental state. The second is sincerity as "singleness of mind;" i.e., integrity and straightforwardness, a mental state with no internal conflicts. Walker maintains that purity undergirds both aspects of sincerity.

Reasoner (1990), an American philosopher, reviews ethics and aesthetics in Western values and classifies sincerity in two categories: external and internal. External sincerity "in an agent is characterized by the correspondence of mental states (beliefs, desires, motivations, intentions) to that which is displayed by the agent to others" (p.473); while internal sincerity "is characterized by agreement between and within currently held mental states" (p.473).

Freud's understanding of sincerity is not so different from these perspectives. Freud uses the term in some writings although he does not enthusiastically pursue the concept as a clinical issue. He applies several meanings to "sincerity," including *openness* (Freud, 1898), *truth-telling* (Freud, 1914), accessibility to one's unconscious mind (Freud, 1920b), and the frankness and straightforwardness that allow one to face psychological pains (Freud, 1905b). In all these examples, *sincerity* describes either an intrapsychic state of mind or a psychological attitude, usually on the patient's side. For Freud, the *sincere* state of mind is one that is not distorted or limited by defensive maneuvers. A patient's *sincere* attitude is one where utterances and behaviors are congruent with each other.

Among post-Freudian thinkers, Meltzer (1971) actively challenges Freud's interpretations of sincerity and insincerity in human relationships. He criticizes Freudian theory from a Kleinian perspective, asserting that the moral and ethical dimensions in Freud's model are confined almost exclusively to an internal object derived from parental super-ego qualities, and that such a model fails to evolve meanings for *sincerity* and *insincerity* in human relationships. Meltzer differentiates between *un*sincerity—a deficit of sincerity and an inability to say what one means which is an expression of infantile mental functioning—and *insincerity,* an incomplete sincerity and inability to mean what one says. Insincerity, he believes, is a perversion derived from a narcissistic structure emerging in the process of moving toward introjective identifications.

Meltzer's analysis, while insightful, remains a developmental process model focused on the patient side. He includes the notion of human relations by following the developmental line of object relationships from infantile structure to narcissistic structure and finally to introjective identifications, but does not refer directly to the ways in which analysts relate to their patients, or how sincerity unfolds in the intersubjective field.

Levenson (1974), a relational thinker, considers sincerity to be relevant to the development of intimacy in an interpersonal relationship. He begins by differentiating between *sincerity* and *authenticity*; the former is described variously as "perfectibility," "purity," or "a state free of stain," which does not necessarily match with one's action. *Authenticity,* the effort to be "oneself, with all its imperfections and shortcomings" (p.363), includes an attempt "to match being and action" (p.363).

In Levenson's model, *sincerity* is an early or primitive form of authenticity. A person knows right and wrong and pursues perfection in his or her mind; but the pursuit is not necessarily reflected in actions, and as a result, it does not have an impact on the interpersonal field. *Authenticity*, however, manifests itself in actions one must take "without sanction or conviction about his rightness or his good intentions" (p.363), and is reflected in the interpersonal field. A mature intimacy, Levenson maintains, evolves in an interpersonal field in which both participants attempt to match their actions and beings, complete with their imperfections and shortcomings.

I believe that Levenson's conception of *sincerity,* while useful, is nonetheless slanted from a Western perspective in two senses: first, his paradigm is premised on the idea that the ethical value is addressed in one's subjectivity; second, that congruence between being and action is the sole criterion of psychological maturity in the interpersonal field. Sincerity in the intersubjective field, however, is an issue of how both participants relate to each other, with each having a limited capacity to say what the field means or mean what the field says, but sharing responsibility for the words and actions provided by the other.

More importantly, from a decolonizing perspective, is that in all these psychoanalytical models the Eastern principle of *makoto* would be seen as a manifestation of an immature mind. *Makoto* ethics allows one to behave in a flexible and even inconsistent manner, without being preoccupied with one's own personal belief. The follower of *makoto* seeks to efface his or her subjectivity, and the congruence of one's being and action has little relevance to ethical development. The *makoto* form of sincerity prioritizes surrender to the "Way of Heaven," and need not always reflect a match of being and action in an individual.

Sincerity in Japanese ethics and aesthetics

Makoto can be interpreted as sincerity, but also as *truthfulness, honesty, genuineness*, or *fidelity*. It was established as a Neo-Confucian moral value, specifically in the Wang Yang-Ming School, in the early modern period in Japan (Sagara, 1980, 1998a). The aesthetic side of *makoto* is emphasized in Japanese culture through many art forms including the way of the warrior, the tea ceremony, and haiku. In business, *makoto* is considered one of the highest moral values, associated with a person who puts their customers' (unspoken) call for human responsibility ahead of their own economic benefit (Ishikawa, 1938; Morita, 2012).

Makoto is based on the theory of "*ji-sho-i*" (time-place-position), whose basic principle is "*shin-seki sabetsu*" (distinguishing between minds and actions). This principle, which was advanced by Tojyu Nakae, a Neo-Confucianist in the 16th century (Sakuma, 1977), is not intended to focus on a Cartesian dualism, but instead conceives of the ethical value of *makoto* as existing beyond any superficial manifestations of personal beliefs and actions. For Tojyu, the ethical value does not necessarily reside in consistency between beliefs and actions or utterances and behavior, but only in purity of mind. Even when people act in opposition to their personal values and beliefs, they are acting ethically as long as their minds reflect a flow that transcends human considerations—in other words, the *cosmos* or *fate*.

This principle of *shin-seki sabetsu* reflects a recognition that human beliefs and actions are ever-changing, depending on time, place, and position. One is directed to seek "the way of being in which one assimilates oneself to the 'Way of Heaven' (mind) without being preoccupied with superficial manifestations of things (action), and allowing oneself to have ever-changing behavior" (Sakuma, 1977, p.30, my translation). *Makoto,* in other words, "is a metaphysical principle which focuses precisely on the relationship between human nature and the Way of Heaven" (Reasoner, 1990, p.483). *Makoto* is not merely a sincere state of mind, but also a reflection of the ever-changing cosmic tide. Like Nature in *Taoism*, this cosmic tide is beyond any individual intention or will, drawing human beings and the Way of Heaven together in the same current, unaffected by any human considerations or artificial controls.

Makoto developed, within Japanese Neo-Confucianism, in reaction to the social class system of the early modern period—the Edo era. At that time, society was defined by four strata or occupational classifications: samurai, peasants, artisans, and merchants. In each stratum, the primary unit of community was the *ie* (household), and the roles of the stratum, *ie*, and the individual within it were all highly circumscribed (Nakane & Oishi, 1990). Although there were some rare and exceptional ways for individuals to change their stratum, it was not easy to challenge the system. The ethic and aesthetic of *makoto* emerged out of the effort to be a human being and recognize one's own feelings *prior* to playing a social role.

Makoto, or *seijitsu,* is considered to be one of the essential virtues of Japanese morality (Watsuji, 1952; Sagara, 1980). The term had its origins in the ancient Shinto idea of "*seimei-shin*" (purity in mind) (Watsuji, 1952), which evolved into a more explicitly moral value, *seichoku* (honesty or uprightness), in the Middle Ages (Watsuji, 1952; Shimokawa, 2001). The term *seichoku* was superseded by *makoto* or "*shisei*" in the early modern period (Sagara, 1980, 1998b).

Watsuji (1952) illustrates the idea of *seimei-shin* through a mythological story, *The Pledge of Amaterasu and Susanoo*, described in the *Kojiki*, or *Records of Ancient Matters*. This story begins with Susanoo being exiled from Heaven because of his violent and malevolent behavior. Accepting this proscription, he goes to *Takamagahara,* located between Heaven and the human world, in order to say goodbye to his sister, Amaterasu. But Amaterasu thinks that Susanoo's aim in coming to *Takamagahara* is to attack Heaven, and when Susanoo arrives, he finds his sister armed against him. Amaterasu insists that Susanoo show his "*seimei-shin,*" the mind of purity, and Susanoo responds by proposing a game of chance. He wins the wager, and Amaterasu admits his victory as evidence of the mind of purity. It is worth noting that this purity is not demonstrated by Susanoo's words or behavior, but by a random outcome, by chance. Watsuji (1952) maintains that this story represents the original form of the Japanese moral value in which purity of mind does not refer to one's following of his or her own maxims, but in surrendering (Ghent, 1990) oneself to the principle of the cosmos. Watsuji concludes that this moral value is derived from a sense of awe towards nature, which is manifested in images of the "savage gods," in ancient nature worship.

Watsuji (1952) emphasizes the connection between a moral value and an aesthetic in *seimei-shin*. He argues that the moral virtue is purity and transparency of mind, and the corresponding evil is dirtiness and turbidity of mind. Purity and transparency are evidence of a selfless mind that reflects an emotional connection to the community one belongs to; dirt and haze are characteristics of a mind stained by a preoccupation with oneself.

Seichoku (honesty or uprightness) is a moral value elaborated in the 14th century in a study of Shinto by Chikafusa Kitabatake. According to Shimokawa (2001), Kitabatake describes *seichoku* as a mind *free-of-stain* which reflects its own rightness like a mirror. For Kitabatake, human nature is like muddy and contaminated water which will, if undisturbed, separate into clear water and lees. *Seichoku* is the pure and transparent aspect of human nature. Only this aspect, which manifests itself in a right and selfless mind, can reflect the cosmic principle. The significant thing is that the cosmic principle is not a maxim or moral imperative, but a principle of change and impermanence.

According to Sagara (1980), the core of Japanese morality was crystalized in the early modern period as *makoto* or *shisei*. Takeuchi (2006) describes this historical development:

> ... since ancient times, Japanese ethics has respected a mind that is open and honest to the other by calling it "a beautiful and bright mind (pure-mind / lit mind)," and disparaged those minds that are hidden and closed to the other by calling them "non-transparent, dirty, dark and foul" (black mind / muddy mind / non-innocent mind). *Wa* (union) of human relationships is always present when people efface the self-minds which create division between them, and relate to each other wholeheartedly with pure minds. The principle of this ethic is not found in an objective norm or order, but in an attitude and pursuit of selflessness and purity of sentiment. Seeking purity in one's individual mind and passionately pursuing *wa* with others had been known as *seichoku mind* until the Middle Ages. It evolved into *makoto*, or *shisei*, after the early modern period, and is currently expressed as *makoto* or *seijitsu*.
>
> *(Takeuchi, 2006, pp.505–506, my translation)*

The Japanese thinkers who elaborated the principle of *makoto* in the early modern period were Neo-Confucianist samurai such as Toju Nakae, Banzan Kumazawa, Jinsai Ito, and Soko Yamaga, and merchants, such as Baigan Ishida. With some differences of emphasis, they all espoused a belief that the basic order of Nature is reflected in human feelings, as opposed to the official view of the Tokugawa government in the Edo era that the basic order of Nature is emulated through perfection and beauty in ritual form and behavior.

I believe that *makoto* is strongly connected to the struggle to live as a human being within a rigid social system. For a samurai such as Banzan, the core of the *makoto* ethic and aesthetic is human feeling and sympathy for those he governs. For Baigan, a merchant, *makoto* requires that even as one pursues profit in one's economic activities, it should be with a pure and selfless mind. And Toju describes *makoto* as an embodiment of the cosmic principle in one's social role. The theory of *ji-sho-i* (time, place, and position), in which personal beliefs and behaviors are seen as ever-changing, regardless of one's role, is the cosmic principle in this social context.

Viewed from a psychoanalytic perspective, *makoto* becomes the analyst's way of encountering patients with a pure mind that reflects the larger flow of the psychoanalytic process over and above personal considerations or professional roles. We know that analysts see patients in order to make a living, advance their professional careers, and realize personal ideals; and *makoto* recognizes that analysts will act out of all these imperatives, sometimes behaving in a ritualistic manner and on other occasions, more spontaneously. An analyst's words and actions may be changeable and inconsistent within a course of psychotherapeutic work, and an analyst may say things that conflict with their personal beliefs, or may not feel their thoughts and feelings as their own. Still, as long as analysts can keep their minds pure and open to the *cosmic tide* of the psychoanalytic process, with all the treasures inherent in psychoanalytic encounters, and remain sensitive to the rhythms of their own and their patients' personal, professional, and societal roles, then, *makoto* says, they can be sincere with their patients, themselves, and their work.

Case vignette

I will examine *makoto* sincerity through a case vignette of Miyuki (also described in Chapter 7), a computer engineer in her late twenties with whom I had worked for eight and a half years. She came to see me complaining of a conflict relationship between her parents.

A notable feature of Miyuki's appearance was a disfigurement caused by a fire at her kindergarten when she was four years old, resulting in keloid scars on the left half of her face. She had undergone multiple plastic surgeries and had learned how to apply make-up skillfully enough that the scarring was not pronounced, yet it was clearly visible to anyone who looked her in the face. When she began treatment, however, Miyuki emphasized that the fundamental conflict she was struggling with was not her appearance, but the way that her parents treated her differently from her siblings. It was disturbing for her that they treated her more delicately than the others and never argued with her.

Miyuki had difficulty talking about her emotional experience. She affected a cheerful and nonchalant air and did not like to show weakness or vulnerability. It took several years for us to work through this reluctance to share her personal feelings. During this process, our talk often revolved around *my* facial expressions, which Miyuki said were open and candid so that she could easily read my emotions and reactions. Through this discussion, she herself came to be more open and honest in session.

Miyuki and I shared an understanding that honesty and openness were of paramount importance to her, and she talked about growing up aware that other people were not being honest or open with her. People said polite things about her appearance in an attempt to spare her pain, but such evasions only made her feel isolated and alienated.

One day, Miyuki surprised me with a question that had long been taboo between us. "I am ugly, aren't I?" she asked. I was not able to reply immediately. "No, you are not ugly" came into my mind, but I did not say it. Other answers came and went—*You don't have to worry about that. What made you ask me about this question now? We should not deny this issue, but I think you are beautiful* – but I said nothing. In fact, I thought that Miyuki was attractive enough, but it is also true that the scarring was prominent on her face. I looked into her eyes. Her serious expression showed that she would not allow me to whitewash my response. There were only a few seconds of silence, but it felt to me like many long minutes. Finally, I could not say anything, but simply and slightly nodded once. She did not reply.

Although she was stunned by my response, and requested that we not talk about my reaction afterward, Miyuki said that after this session she grew less nervous and anxious. Toward the end of her therapy, Miyuki felt comfortable enough to talk openly about painful experiences and events that had occurred in her life, and her openness helped me to engage with her vulnerability and weakness. Ultimately, she was able to tell me, "I was shocked by your confirmation of my word. But it was good because you were honest. People always try to be nice, but it is a lie … that was a moment of honesty and it made me feel better about my life."

If we accept that I was sincere in a *makoto* sense in this interaction, what was the fundamental element of this sincerity? Was it in my openness and honesty? Careful reading of this case vignette suggests that the answer is no. Although Miyuki said that I was honest, in fact, I was not. I did not simply think that she was ugly; I did not give any verbal answer to her question except for a nod; I failed to share many thoughts that were in my mind; I did not express my thoughts and feelings completely nor did they match my actions.

Makoto, in this case, cannot be understood as the sincerity that Meltzer (1971) describes. From his perspective, my nod would be seen as ersatz wisdom delivered in an insincere fashion, and Miyuki's not replying to my nod as her unsincere effort to avoid facing her pain. Neither can this be understood as the sincerity or authenticity that Levenson (1974) posits. My nodding was neither an effort to pursue perfectibility or purity of my mind, nor was it an example of matching being and action. In the moment of nodding, my mind was a welter of thoughts and emotions in conflict with one another. Nodding was not an action matched to my subjectivity or conviction; but an act that happened to appear in the moment when my preoccupation with my own thoughts, intentions, and feelings disappeared.

Makoto in this case can be understood as surrendering myself to the cosmic tide of the universe, which can be seen as the irrationality of the world and human vulnerability. In this dimension, all personal and professional considerations were let go, and I was not thinking about myself or Miyuki. The nodding was less my own action than an element of the intersubjective field.

Discussion and conclusion

This case vignette suggests that, in seeking sincerity in psychoanalytic practice, the issue is not always whether or not a person's utterances and actions are consistent or congruent with each other. Sincerity, in *makoto* terms, is rather an issue of how both participants can efface their preoccupation with social and professional roles. By doing so, they are able to feel the cosmic tide of a psychoanalytic process prior to the awareness of their being and roles.

What is the *cosmic tide of a psychoanalytic process*? I believe that, at the core, it is the contingency of human encounter. In Japanese cosmology, all human encounters are in the hands of a "god at play" (Obama, 2006; Togashi, 2014a). This god did not create the laws of the world, nor does he judge a person's behavior. The god has no purposes or ideals, and he plays dice with no particular aim except for the sake of playing. The god at play does not provide a reason why a person is born, why she is exposed to traumatic events, or why she encounters the person she loves. The cosmic tide of random events precedes any given human interaction; similarly, the cosmic tide of a therapeutic process has also been prepared before an analyst and a patient meet each other.

The randomness of the world creates human vulnerability and radical loneliness. In its irrationality, we find ourselves suffering and causing suffering without rational reasons. What my nodding enacted in the relationship with Miyuki was my human feeling for the contingency of our encounter. Until the moment when she asked me if she was ugly, I had felt guilty about *not* having scars on *my* face. I separated us into categories of *traumatized* and *non-traumatized*, and by doing so I denied the shared cruelty and impermanence of the world.

When Miyuki asked me if she was ugly, I had to face the fact that it could have been me who had the scars on my face; that it was totally random and coincidental that it was she who was exposed to that traumatic event. Simultaneously, I came to recognize the ultimate impossibility of understanding her pain. Of course, I attempted to understand; I tried to imagine how painful her life had been, and I tried to envision how my life would have been changed if I'd had her scars on my face. But in the end, I had to admit that it was impossible for me to sense her pain at all; I had to accept the radical incommensurability between us—through which, ironically, we could become equally human. It was at that moment that my nod happened to appear in this therapeutic process. All therapeutic constellations were aggregated in that nod, at that particular place and time.

The concept of *makoto* sheds fresh light on our understanding of intersubjective processes. As the example of my work with Miyuki indicates, *makoto* is a sincerity that is informed by our sense of being human among other human beings. The *ethical value* of *makoto* informs a creative moment in which both participants encounter each other as human beings beyond their radical incommensurability; the *aesthetic* of *makoto* allows for a creative space in which both participants are seen as a part of the cosmos. Pursuing the ethical value and aesthetic of *makoto* keeps both participants human at the moment when they meet each other in social and professional services.

4

THE MOTIVATIONAL SYSTEM OF MOVING TOWARD ZERO

Emptiness is a moment without context, in which there are no distinctions made between self and other, between a suffering patient and an analyst acting within a professional role, between right and wrong. It is the moment before and beyond artificially named differences. It is an aspect of Nature emerging in analytic work, from which everything is born and to which everything is reduced.

How is emptiness manifested in therapeutic process? It is the therapeutic phenomenon in which all possibilities of clinical transformation reside, and we can refer to it as the *zero moment*, in which all therapeutic actions are cancelled out, from which any meaning of therapeutic process emerges and into which they flit away. As discussed in the Preface, the *zero* is not one individual moment; temporally, it can be manifested in a split second in a session, a whole session, or a ten-year analysis. A therapeutic dialogue, therefore, can be seen as a succession of *zero moments*, inclusive of every possibility and continually creating context, moment by moment. But unless we are aware of it, the moment remains invisible, hidden within the context that the moment itself creates.

In this chapter, I will explore a clinical manifestation of the zero moment from the perspective of motivational systems theory (Lichtenberg, 1988, 1989, 2001; Lichtenberg & Kindler, 1994; Lichtenberg, Lachmann, & Fosshage, 1992, 1996, 2011; Fosshage, 1995) and attempt to illustrate the notion of *emptiness* within a Western psychoanalytic model. Returning to the case vignette from Chapter 1, I explore the ways in which the zero moment emerges and develops in a human relationship, and demonstrate how the partners in an analytic dyad, by transcending their personal preoccupations, can surrender to this process and recover a sense of being human.

A sleeping lady

It was approximately three months after beginning her psychoanalysis that I found that my patient, Yukiko, had fallen asleep on the couch. She had been talking about an art project she was devoting herself to, and I had attempted to explore her narrative: what made her choose this project; why did she want to talk about it in this particular session; how did she experience the colleagues she worked with?

After I ran through these queries, I tried to present my understanding of the connection between her devotion to the project and her psychological history, but in the midst of my explanation, I heard a slight sound of her breathing. I stopped talking and listened, trying to understand what was going on. Was she asleep? Or pretending to sleep?

"Yukiko?" I said. No answer but the sound of her sleeping breath. I asked myself, "What is this? Is she tired today? Is my interpretation boring her? Is she resistant to listening to my comments?"

I was puzzled. Despite the noisy questions in my mind, I couldn't say anything. I let her sleep for five minutes or so. I could hear her breathing, and she looked happy.

As I described in Chapter 1, Yukiko was a photographer in her early thirties who entered psychoanalysis in order to deal with her fear of intimacy. Yukiko was the only child of a mother with minor paranoid tendencies and a self-absorbed and indifferent father. Her mother maintained that all people in the world operate with malicious intent. She claimed, "If a person is nice to you, be careful. They only seek to plunge you into darkness."

Yukiko was psychoanalytically inclined and elected to embark on a four-times a week psychoanalysis on the couch. For the first three months, she had been an active and responsive patient, vividly providing associations, histories, and emotional experiences from her private and professional life. She enjoyed talking about the ideas in her art projects, which in turn inspired me. Although I wondered why no concrete human figures showed up in her narratives or dreams, I felt that she was a dream patient. But I was soon to find that her sessions would not be so easy.

For the first few months after she began falling asleep, I attempted to deal with her behavior through standard psychoanalytic procedures. Lying on the couch, Yukiko usually began by talking for five to ten minutes about something she was interested in. I would carefully listen to her talk and then provide some comments, at which point I would find that she had fallen asleep. I would wake her up and tell her that she had asleep, and she would always ask, "Really? I fell asleep?"

"Yes. You have been completely asleep. What do you think might make you fall asleep every session? Do you have any ideas?"

"Well, maybe I am tired?"

"I believe that we need to explore this more carefully. You come to my office four times a week and every session you fall asleep in the middle of our talk. Do you have any problems with my understandings or comments?"

"No, I don't think that I have any problems with you."

"It seems to me that your falling asleep has to do with your fear of intimacy. You see me four times a week here and lie on the couch; you are asked to talk about your personal experiences. In other words, you and I have an emotionally close relationship … Can you hear me? Yukiko?" And I would find that she had fallen asleep again.

Although I was baffled by her sleeping, I did not experience the episodes as unpleasant; the scene often brought a smile to my face. Still, I began to feel that all my efforts were being negated or disregarded. I was desperate to analyze the meaning of Yukiko's sleep at any cost and had run through numerous influences and theories. This situation continued for almost a year.

The biggest problem for us during this time was that Yukiko experienced a deflation of her professional creativity. She claimed that she could not reach the essential part of her artistic sensitivity. To me, this phenomenon seemed related to her sleeping, but either Yukiko would not allow me to explore the meaning of that, or she could not stop sleeping even if she wanted to deal with the issue with me. I was desperately worried about her professional career, and I felt helpless and powerless as an analyst.

In my efforts to make sense of Yukiko's behavior, I finally hit upon what I felt was an apt description: she was in a "cocoon state," in which she withdrew from the outside world, including me, by shutting down all stimuli. When I reached this understanding, I was able to create some space in my thoughts. I no longer rushed to analyze and prevent her sleeping. I let her sleep as long as she wanted, typically about thirty minutes. Sitting behind the couch, I spent the time alone and listened to her breathing. On most occasions, I did not do anything during her periods of slumber. I could have read a book or a paper, but I preferred to let myself drift without paying attention to anything. Extremely quiet hours went by in our sessions. Yukiko usually woke up almost precisely five minutes before each session ended, and always asked me if she had been asleep. I simply answered, "Yes." She always looked mildly surprised, and said, "Really?" Then she ended the session and left my office smiling at me.

It was about a year after I began characterizing her sleeping as a "cocoon state" that Yukiko herself said, "It is weird that I fall asleep every session. Almost a whole session." She continued, "I'm sorry, but when I am here, I cannot resist falling asleep." Around the same time, she said that her creativity had come back to her. She began working hard and actively devoting herself to the photo business.

My query about what made her sleep

What was Yukiko's sleep? What was our work during this period? Even after we terminated analysis, I often remembered and reflected on it.

First, I asked myself if Yukiko was really in a *cocoon state*. Although it is true that this phrase was quite useful to me, helping me to stay with Yukiko in my therapeutic office without rushing to analyze, my answer is no. Even when she was asleep, she was not totally removed; she maintained some awareness of time. She always woke up exactly five minutes before the end of a session. She seemed to listen to my voice, and she could talk with me immediately after I woke her up.

Did Yukiko physiologically regulate herself into this state in order to reduce external stimuli? Was she withdrawing from the relationship with me at the cost of attachment? Did she develop an aversive relationship with me? My answer to all of these queries is, "Yes, all these descriptions are true in one sense or another, but ..."

After deep contemplation, I came to recognize that I was missing the whole point, which was not how Yukiko was when she slept, but how *I* was. For it was not Yukiko who struggled with this analytic relationship, but myself. The conflict did not appear in her, but in me. In a certain sense, she was stable. Her answer was always clear and consistent; whatever I did, she fell asleep. The key factor in this condition was what was happening in me, and how my psychological process influenced our analytic relationship.

During the first few months of this period, I actively tried to explore Yukiko's behavior and psychological state. I urged her to understand what might be making her sleep and what the basic motive for this behavior was. I was anxious and uncomfortable because I felt that I was being negated by her. I rushed to analyze and interpret her periods of sleep. Using a standard psychoanalytic or self psychological approach, I tried to help her to talk without falling asleep, expecting to resolve the underlying issue and feel myself a skilled analyst. But all my efforts failed. Whenever I tried to articulate her sleep through a standard analytic approach, she immediately fell asleep again.

What changed this impasse was my surrender (Ghent, 1990) to this circumstance. I stopped thinking, exploring, analysing, and focusing on her through a psychoanalytic perspective, and only tried to be present. My arousal level and my overall physiological state lowered. I did not feel anything.

It was not easy for me to maintain this state. As a psychoanalyst, I was trained to explore the meaning of my patients' behavior. Even if a patient falls asleep, this is behavior that I am driven to analyze and understand. But I was forced to recognize that the heightening of my thoughts, feelings, intimacy, interest, and sensuality had only resulted in the deflation of Yukiko's creativity.

Lichtenberg (2009) suggests five areas of inquiry to help an analyst explore and describe the psychological process of an observed event. He states:

> What *influences* have bearing on the emergence and unfolding of this event? What *motives and intentions* are dominant, participating, conflicting, or dormant? What *inferences* does the individual draw from current and past similar events, what conscious and unconscious belief systems have evolved from those inferences, and what expectations guide future perceptions and assumptions? What are the *modes of communication*—gestural, facial, verbal, relational, and behavioral, either implicit or explicit—that inform individuals about themselves and others, and tell others about them? What are the means and effects of *regulation* of affect, cognition, and behavior? Based on their theoretical orientation and their response to the specific event under consideration, analysts will ascribe differing significance to factors of influence, motivation, inference, communication, and regulation.
>
> *(Lichtenberg, 2009, p. 421; italics in original)*

As a trained psychoanalyst, these perspectives infiltrate every aspect of my thoughts, but I had to give them up. And indeed, when I finally relinquished my analytic mindset, Yukiko's creativity came back to her.

As I described in Chapter 1, Yukiko described her way of photographing an object by saying that she always "waited for a moment of *nothingness*" when she shot. According to her, she "vanished" her self-consciousness at the very moment when she shot. She said that she could not capture the essence of nature and her human subjects if even a tiny piece of "I" slid into her consciousness.

Despite her eloquent description, I did not think that Yukiko really "vanished" herself at a moment of nothingness, for she was motivated to shoot the picture and never forgot to press the shutter button. By the same token, I would not say that Yukiko attempted to "vanish" herself by falling asleep. As I described earlier, she maintained a sense of time, and, at a certain level, kept communicating with me. Nor do I think that I attempted to vanish myself by stopping my psychoanalytic thoughts. What we did at that time, in my understanding, was to stay in the moment in which all psychological and interactive processes were still, balanced, and regulated at a low level.

I do not deny that Yukiko's sleep indicated her avoidance of the development of an intimate relationship. But the idea of an "avoidance," in itself, includes the notion that "something" should have been there. Claiming that Yukiko avoided intimacy implies the analyst's effort to search for intimacy. I would like to emphasize here that Yukiko's and my great interest was not in how *something* emerges in a space of nothingness, but how *everything emerges at the same time* in an analytic relationship, with psychological and interactive processes cancelling one another out.

A silent lady

Even after she stopped sleeping on the couch in session, Yukiko often had periods of silence, frequently for minutes at a time. When I asked her to tell me how she felt during these silences, her reply was ambiguous; "I don't know. My mind was just absent." Her silence looked, without question, like a typical example of therapeutic resistance, indicating that there was some transference behind it.

I treated this silence carefully, to avoid making her fall asleep again. I tried not to explore it as actively as I might have done, and I allowed her to make time for silence. My efforts appeared to be successful. Yukiko enjoyed talking about anything, as long as I gave less focus to her silence, and she was delighted when her artistic sensitivity came back to her. Still, it was not so easy for me to distract my attention from these quiet periods.

Yukiko was very sensitive to my state of mind. If my interest and attention moved toward her psychological state, she immediately recognized it and said, "What are you thinking about?" When this happened, she often fell into a dream state or changed topics. The development of a sense of intimacy, attachment, caregiving, or any search for optimal distance by me led to the same result. If I allowed myself to go forward in a particular direction or intention—even a single step—she seemed to feel uncomfortable. During this period, I simply tried to be with her, keeping my arousal and physiological state at a low level. As long as I kept myself in this state, she also stayed calm and felt easy.

Yukiko gradually felt more comfortable being with others. Although she did not have very many intimate relationships, she now had some good friendships in her professional life. She was no longer as afraid of being betrayed or used by others as she had been. She developed a good reputation in her field.

As she devoted herself to professional activity more, she frequently talked to me about her work and often brought in examples. She showed me a series of photos she had shot which made it clear to me that she liked to shoot human beings, despite her bashfulness. The people in the pictures were dynamic and powerful, vivid and extremely expressive. She said "I like to shoot awesome nature, such as mountains and rivers, but I like humans more. My job is to capture the rhythm of life in people."

In one session, Yukiko talked about a short trip made with a male colleague at a web company's request. She was nervous and felt uncomfortable being with him for the whole day. She said, "I know it was just for a day, not so long a time. But it was too long for me. He is not a bad person, but I felt strange. I wish I could have traveled by myself. Maybe I want to concentrate on my job. I don't like myself feeling distressed by such a small issue. I know that it is important for me to keep good relations with colleagues and I have tried. Indeed, it was not so bad for me to be with him. I enjoyed chatting with him and talking about photography. He is a really professional person who I can respect. Still, I need time by myself in order to concentrate and be able to do my job."

As she began to talk, I found my brain working very hard. What was it she wanted to say through this episode? Was she expressing an essential conflict? What did she expect me to say? How did she want to communicate with me through this story? How did she feel about me during her speech?

I organized some hypotheses for each issue and attempted to articulate the priority for each moment: intimacy with others; trust; a conflict around career pursuits; or a yearning to share some feeling with me. Usually my mind works harder and harder toward the end of a patient's relating, processing what I'm hearing until I feel the moment is right to make comments. In Yukiko's case, however, toward the end of her story my thoughts slowed down and stopped as she finished. There was no motivation in me to ask a question or make a comment. Instead, there was a pause. The pause was a very short, but our communication and my internal activities were both suspended; probably her internal activities went down, too.

In this pause I did not feel anything and stayed with her without doing anything. Yukiko did not struggle to deal with the pause. She sometimes continued to talk and sometimes gave me her interpretation of her feelings. And often, she remained quiet for a while. In other words, our relationship was organized around the pause.

It was four years after the beginning of Yukiko's psychoanalysis that she was offered a good position in a large company in another city and had to leave town. There were many issues to explore: what made her decide to get this position even though she knew that she would have to leave our town? What did she expect would happen in a new city? What did it mean to her that we would separate? How did she want to terminate her analysis? What did she want to say at the final session? How did she experience her analysis with me?

I asked Yukiko a few times to tell me how she felt about termination. She answered only once, "I am okay now. I feel sad, though." We did not turn to this issue very often but enjoyed talking about her photos. At the very end of the analysis, she said, "Thank you. I feel confident in myself as a photographer."

Discussion and conclusion

Motivational system for moving toward zero

Motivational systems theory is a psychoanalytic model in contemporary self-psychology. The basic idea was laid out in the 1980s by Joseph Lichtenberg, and elaborated by Lichtenberg, Lachmann and Fosshage (Lichtenberg, 1988, 1989, 2001; Lichtenberg & Kindler, 1994; Lichtenberg, Lachmann, & Fosshage, 1992, 1996, 2011; Fosshage, 1995). The theory describes how a human being is motivated in a particular direction from a dynamic systems view. It also fits, they maintain (Lichtenberg, Lachmann, & Fosshage, 2011), within complexity theory.

In this model, the motivational systems consist of seven goals and intentions, five fundamental information processing systems, and two linking processes to mediate between them. The seven goals and intentions are: 1) physiological regulation; 2) attachment to individuals; 3) affiliation with groups; 4) caregiving; 5) exploration and assertion of preferences and capacities; 6) sensuality and sexuality; and 7) aversive responses of antagonism and withdrawal. They each imply a direction and a goal towards which an individual is motivated to move. The fundamental information processing systems which combine with the motivational systems are perception, cognition, affect, memory, and recursive awareness. They are linked by two imagistic and linguistic symbolic processes: affect and metaphor.

Unlike Freud's instinctual drive theory, motivational systems theory is not a categorical map for determining a single motivation. Rather, it is a set of dynamic systems which "provides a way to view each human as an individual, the manner in which changes occurs, and the dissemination and transfer of information" (Lichtenberg, Lachmann, & Fosshage, 2011, p.3). They spelled out this model as follows:

> First, each individual can be thought of as a separate *open* system (a self-system) comprised of multiple, also open, subsystems (multiple motivational systems) ... Second, the perturbation in any system may diminish under some conditions or rise to a tipping point after which the trajectory of the system is

> altered ... Third, complex systems require the recognition, storage, accessibility, and transmission of information to be able to adapt to changing conditions in their environment.
>
> *(Lichtenberg, Lachmann, & Fosshage, 2011, p.3;* italics *in original)*

The motivation systems theory helps a clinician to follow a psychoanalytic interaction, which changes, moment by moment, in complex ways. At a particular time, one system and one information process will be in the foreground and the others in the background; at another, a system which was background a few seconds ago comes to the fore. Motivational systems are multi-tiered and polyphonic, and development of the systems is non-linear. The dynamic changing of motivation systems in each person affects others in human interactions, and the relational system also alters moment by moment under their influence.

In this model, when Yukiko falls into silence, we could say that motivational systems of *physiological regulation* and *aversive responses of antagonism and withdrawal* are in the foreground, yet the systems of attachment and *exploration and assertion of preferences and capacities* do not stop working. They continue, but in the background. Yukiko kept communicating with me, at a certain level, and kept exploring her mind and mine. My motivational systems were also affected by and affecting Yukiko's systems, and our relational systems were co-created in this interaction.

Using this model, how should we describe the moment in which Yukiko and I stopped actively exploring our psychological processes? First, Yukiko was asleep, next we were in silence, and finally we created a pause. As described in the case vignette, we did not stop interacting with each other or allow ourselves to vanish. Even when she was asleep, we kept interacting at a certain level, although our interaction was severely impaired. Our motivational systems were regulated at a low level but maintained a balance. No motivational system was salient in this context, and the systems became, on the whole, still and quiet. We could call this a motivational system moving toward zero.

Moving toward zero is not an intention or a goal, but an attribute of the whole complex system, which becomes critical in a transient period at the border between stability and chaos. Moving toward zero is not a nirvana principle (Freud, 1920a), because it does not refer to a mental life's "effort to reduce, to keep constant or to remove internal tension due to stimuli" (pp.54–55). It is not the death instinct (Freud, 1920a, 1923a, 1924) either, because it does not refer to a psychological drive "to lead organic life back into the inanimate state" (Freud, 1923b, p.40) as opposed to the libidinal drive urging survival and creation.

Within this transient moment, the analyst's (and probably also the patient's) preoccupation with his or her identity, sense of self, and his or her professional, therapeutic, social, and cultural roles fades away. Yukiko's case history is a vivid example of what an analytic couple's surrendering themselves to emptiness looks like. During the whole process, they are always analyst and patient, communicating with each other in many dimensions. But moment by moment, they are freed from their preoccupation with artificially named differences and roles and are able to stay within the larger flow and rhythms of the therapeutic process.

Sincerity, surrender, and zero

A motivational system for moving toward zero does not extinguish or remove anything from the analytic relationship. Rather it creates something. In Yukiko's case, as all motivational systems moved toward zero, the therapist reached a kind of sincerity or authenticity; and Yukiko accessed the essential aspect of her artistic creativity, which allowed her to share the "it-ness" or core of aesthetics of nature, and finally human beings. I believe that both of us shared these experiences with each other.

I believe that *makoto* sincerity exists in this therapeutic dialogue and interaction, for it is the sense of sincerity and aesthetics of nature and human beings that are, as discussed in Chapter 3, the core element of *makoto*. Both participants are together simply as human beings, as the "therapeutic" relationship dwindles to zero. This entails their surrendering to emptiness.

It is no wonder that this moment emerged between Yukiko and I, for she needed a sincerity that she could indulge in fully, in contrast to the paranoid perspective given by her mother. What dissolved the analytic impasse in Yukiko's case was our surrender to the "moment of nothingness," as she called it. By stopping thinking, exploring, analyzing, and focusing on her psychological condition, we surrendered ourselves to the relational system, which moved to a calm state of stillness.

What is sincere and what is insincere in this relationship? One may say that Yukiko was not sincere; according to Meltzer's (1971) model, she was not able to say what she really meant and remained in an infantile preverbal state of mind by shutting down all communication with me. One may also say that the original efforts of her analyst *were* sincere. He tackled the problem of her sleeping head-on and sought language to create unity in her mind.

However, once we define sincerity and insincerity as unfolding in the intersubjective field, we may say that Yukiko *was* sincere and her analyst *not* sincere at the beginning of her analysis. The interaction between Yukiko and her analyst was organized around the question of whether there can be an uncontaminated space in human relationships. Yukiko was not able to resist falling asleep, and her analyst was not able to stop her sleeping. The intersubjective process went on to highlight the genuineness or pure essence of their relationship, one beyond their control. Yukiko was sincere in that her sleeping genuinely reflected her essence; her analyst was not sincere because he rejected involvement with this essence due to his preoccupation with resolving it.

Both participants finally stopped controlling the field through their customary personal, professional, and social thoughts, and allowed themselves to stay with the pure essence of the relationship. They effaced their personal preoccupations, and the analytic process became a sincere one. The essence of human interaction emerged in this intersubjective field and made Yukiko feel herself as being human in this world.

The ethical dimension of sincerity is reflected in the analyst's responding to the call for responsibility from the intersubjective field. The aesthetic dimension of sincerity is shown by the analyst becoming a faithful witness to the analytic relationship. Abandoning private or idiosyncratic visions, he witnessed the relationship, reflected it in himself, and surrendered to it. The effort itself reified purity, brightness, and uprightness in the field.

This is the moment of *makoto*/sincerity we have discussed elsewhere (Brothers & Togashi, 2019). As discussed in Chapter 3, *makoto* sincerity is informed by our sense of being human, and only the human relationship remains in the therapeutic dialogue and interaction. Both participants are together only as people, and the "therapeutic" relationship comes to zero.

5

TRAUMA, CONTINGENCY, AND THE PSYCHOANALYTIC ZERO

During my psychoanalytic training in New York, one of the biggest issues for my personal analysis was my phobia of one picture—a photo of a little girl in Hiroshima in 1945, who looked into the lens of the camera with empty eyes. The black and white picture showed the girl surrounded by burnt-out ruins; one precious life that had survived the atomic bomb. She showed no emotions, no feelings, and no fears. Her blankness was burned into my brain and seeing her image in my dreams often woke me up in the middle of the night.

In childhood, I was made to see many movies and photos of the Second World War at school and at home. Many of them were grotesque dead bodies and burned human faces. One day I encountered the little girl's photo. It did not look as horrible as the others; she was alive, with no visible injury. I could have found some hope in her picture, but what I felt instead was a deep fear and guilt. The photo was a symbol of my crime, my vulnerability, my craziness, and my victimization. Why was I so scared of seeing the photo? Who was she?

My late father was born in 1944. He was a committed activist during the student movement of the 1960s, fighting riot police throughout most of his college years. He disapproved of many aspects of his country and was especially critical of Japanese imperialism during the Second World War. Since my youngest years, he had taught me about Japan's actions during the Great War and forced me to view photos and movies of the destruction caused by the Great Tokyo Air Raid and the atomic bombs in Hiroshima and Nagasaki. I remember him shouting at me, "This is our crime. This is our sin," but only in reference to photos of dead or injured Japanese people. I do not remember him saying anything about other nationalities, whose countries were mercilessly invaded and bombarded by the Japanese army and navy before and during the Second World War. His twisted logic confused me. Who was I in these photos? Was I the victimizer or a victim? I have asked myself these questions many times in the years since but found no answer.

I knew that my paternal grandfather had been in Manchuria in the 1940s as a soldier in a mounted unit, although I knew nothing more in detail. After the war, he came home to Japan and became a police officer. A few days after my grandfather's funeral, when I was in junior high school, it occurred to me to wonder if there might have been some connection between my father's strong beliefs and my grandfather's military life. I asked relatives what my grandfather had said about the Great War, and how my father had talked about that period in his life, but my inquiries revealed nothing. No one had ever heard either of them speak about the war. My grandfather never talked about what he did in China and it seemed that no one had ever asked him what he saw there. It had been a taboo, not an incest taboo, but an intersubjective one (Togashi, 2016a). So, was my grandfather a victimizer or victim? What about my father? Who were they?

'Human' condition and trauma

It is widely known that early in the history of psychoanalysis, trauma was not a reputable term in the psychoanalytic community. In the last two decades, however, there has been a reaction to this tradition and psychoanalysts have become more open to considering the role of trauma in human suffering (Huppertz, 2018). Relational groups, who deny "the myth of the isolated mind" (Stolorow & Atwood, 1992; Stolorow & Atwood, 1994), place particular value on the idea of trauma.

Intersubjective theorists have emphasized that trauma is always and already a part of the historical, cultural, and social context in which it occurs (Stolorow & Atwood, 1992; Stolorow, 2007). They contend that all trauma can be called "epistemological trauma," in that "the effect of such a trauma is the shattering of confidence in one's own mind" (Atwood, 2011, p.396). Although these are useful insights, this conception of trauma is still grounded in a Western perspective. When psychoanalysts refer to trauma, especially societal trauma caused by wars, natural disasters, and crimes, they implicitly claim that *something not-me* is wrong and that *something not-me* shatters something important *in me.* Their perspective includes, in itself, dichotomies and distinctions made between something which destroys me and the *me* who is destroyed; or between a well-functioning mind, before something happened and a malfunctioning mind as a result of something happening. This chapter examines trauma from a non-Western perspective, drawing on my own Asian cultural background, which rejects such differences.

Once we say that trauma is situated in an historical, cultural, and social context, we have to say that trauma *is* a human life, for emotional life in this context is no longer seen as an object that can be destroyed by something *not-me.* There are many types of traumatic events—natural disaster, war, social injustice, genocide, abuse, sexual violence, and other crimes—and the emotions that accompany them are destroyers as well as destroyed. A traumatic experience not only shatters human emotional experience but also *is* human emotional experience.

My understanding of trauma is influenced by *Taoism*, a philosophical tradition of Chinese origin that understands human suffering very differently from a Western view. *Taoism* presupposes the existence of *Tao*, the Way, the indefinable principle of the universe which is a reflection and manifestation of Nature. In *Taoism*, Nature is a dynamically continuous flow, infinitely changing and moving, and involving all aspects of being in the universe, a universe that has neither abstractions nor names. In this universe, there are no distinctions and all contradictions are resolved. Absence means being; being means absence. "Destroyer" is also "destroyed." *Taoists*, despite differences between particular schools, generally emphasize effortless action, "naturalness," and "spontaneity" which entails surrendering themselves to the nameless universe.

A human being attempts to avoid surrendering him or herself to the nameless universe by controlling and "naming" the world. A person attempts to prevent, escape, or understand the irrationality of a traumatic event by discovering its mechanism, making the trauma visible by naming its human condition. But in such efforts, the trauma creates suffering and shatters the person. One of my patients, who lost a beloved wife in a traffic accident, was preoccupied with the idea that, "I could have prevented the accident," and so tortured himself.

For *Taoists*, it is this human capacity for preoccupation—going against the flow of *Tao*—that creates a world of wounds and suffering. For them, "human life is a life of misery and a sad delusion" (Møllgaard, 2007, p.18) and the human life is trauma itself. In the human world's need for names and categories, *Tao* is divided and dichotomies emerge. "Not big" means "small," "not ugly" means "beautiful," and "not suffering" means "peace." Such is the "human" condition, the artificial "world that results in the neglect of the world qua world" (Møllgaard, 2007, p.17).

When a person fails to surrender to the nameless universe, they find themselves in the "human" traumatic world. Trauma, in this paradigm, is neither a human experience nor an actual event, but simply what a human life is, a life that becomes visible in the act of naming.

At this point, it is important to differentiate *trauma* from *traumatization*. The former is human life itself. Trauma creates the human world—including human suffering and anguish—but it does not necessarily lead to pathology or mental problems. Trauma can make a person aware of being in a particular world and awakens this awareness with powerful emotional impact. Without trauma, people would neither be able to see what the human world is like, nor play a role in the world.

Traumatization, on the other hand, is a psychological state in which a human mind or community is divided, and which creates mental illnesses in both individuals and communities. A traumatized person or community is preoccupied with division, identifying themselves as either "us" or "them," (Brothers, 2008; Togashi & Kottler, 2019) and dividing the world into "those who experienced it" and "those who did not," "those who were there" and "those who were not there," and "victim" and "victimizer." A person who is traumatized immediately gets busy identifying him or herself with a side.

I do not mean to suggest that a person who is not traumatized lives only in the nameless universe; he or she lives in the "human" world, with names and categories, as well. No one can fully escape from human preoccupations; no one avoids the temptation to organize the world by naming others, his environment, and him or herself. And yet, one is not *always naming*. A person who is not traumatized can, from time to time, give him or herself completely to the nameless universe. A traumatized person, by contrast, remains trapped in human division.

My late father was preoccupied with controlling history and society. He accused the Japanese people of crimes by describing those who were deeply wounded and bombarded by the atomic bombs. His confusing expression regarding the Second World War indicated that he was trapped between identifying with victims and victimizers, justice and injustice, and remained trapped in this oscillation through his entire lifetime. He positioned himself as a perpetrator; but behind the name which trapped him for his entire life, there was another name, *victim*, which remained unspoken. His discourse was always twisted, because he was a victimized perpetrator.

The minds of my entire family, including my late grandfather, were divided between events that could be spoken about and those which could not. The same can be said of Japanese society, culture, and our country. Japanese people often speak of their history as if it were separated into two different times—before and after the Great War—although they know that they make up one continuous history. Many people who were born before the Great War continued their lives during and after, yet they find it impossible to connect the two divided worlds. The names we use, "prewar" and "postwar," divide the universe and create a world in which the two can never be brought together. It is precisely in this sense that I can say that my grandfather, my father, and I have been traumatized; and my family and society—in fact, all Asian people, our countries and the times that we live in—have been traumatized, too.

How do we tell the victim from the victimizer, or tell who is on the side of justice or injustice? Picture a former Nazi who lives fifty years hidden away in a small town, certain that government or vigilante Nazi hunters are seeking him, jumping at shadows and fearing every knock on the door—is he a victim or victimizer? Similarly, consider the Japanese medical officer who suffers chronic depression and nightmares and was never able to resume practicing medicine after the war because he participated in the production of biological weapons—victim or victimizer? Is the employee of the doomed nuclear plant in Fukushima during the Great East Japan Earthquake[1] a victim or a victimizer?

We cannot answer these questions. None of these lives can be confined to such categorizations. It is coincidental that this person worked for the nuclear plant. Had he or she been born in a different place, or simply been rejected at a job interview, his or her life would have been completely different. The *Tao*, the nameless universe, makes no distinction between victim or victimizer, accuser or accused, perpetrator or sufferer. Such distinctions belong to the material world, and once traumatized, you are confined to one side or other of the divide.

In saying that trauma is human life itself, I mean that trauma is the *zero point* from which the state of our being is born and to which it is reduced (Togashi, 2017d, 2017g). *Zero* is neither the nameless universe nor emptiness, but it is the original touch point between a person and the world that has yet to be named, a world without categories. Although people are divided once they are traumatized, there are no divisions or categories *at the moment of traumatization*. Categories emerge *after* the trauma is visible and *named*. Before the trauma, a person might become anything: victim, victimizer, or non-participating bystander. They might survive or die.

Before the atomic bomb exploded over Hiroshima, no one could tell who would or would not be a survivor. Even regarding the pilot who dropped the bomb, it could not be said that his role was entirely *of his own choosing;* he might just as easily have been deployed in the European theater of war rather than the Asian, in the Navy rather than the Army Air Corps. Everything is subject to chance (Togashi, 2014a, 2014b).

I am not saying that a victim is a perpetrator. There is no question about the victimization of a person who is raped, abused, or tortured. I am saying that a victim could have been a perpetrator in another setting, just as a perpetrator could have been a victim in other circumstances. In the nameless universe, no one can say who might be a victim and who can be a perpetrator.

Nor am I saying that we are not responsible for what we do, but rather, paradoxically perhaps, I am claiming that we cannot deny our responsibility for *any* action *because* everything is coincidental. In other words, at the zero point of trauma, everyone is both player and witness. Like a "black hole/white hole" dyad, trauma is the origin point of the human world. It creates traumatization, of course, but also creates everything in the human world. Traumatized people, like my family, lose the infinite potential of the world by confining it to a certain form.

How can we heal our traumatization and make the confined and limited world open again for infinite growth potential? My answer is, if traumatization is based on naming and categorization, and naming and categorization creates suffering and destroys human potential, it is our responsibility to surrender ourselves to the nameless or category-less world—to become *player-witnesses* (*toji-sha*, in Japanese) in this traumatic world and take responsibility for our being. The player-witness is not a person who simply witnesses an event, but a person who knows that, under other circumstances, he or she could have taken any role, in that event or any other. When we stay in the divided world, we objectify and abstract ourselves and those belonging to not-our-side: "They are people who perpetrated war-crimes, but I am not;" "They were killed in the earthquake, but I was not;" and "They are unjust, but I am just." We may claim that we could not be a Hitler, that we are different from him, and disavow the part of ourselves which might have been a Hitler. But that part still exists and, under other circumstances, in another universe, we could be Hitler.

Human life is tragic. No one can resist the world's contingency. But if we allow ourselves to see that contingency, we can recognize that people are not categories, and everyone contains the potential to be victim, victimizer or bystander. In the potential field, there are no sides and we are all player-witnesses of the world.

In the psychoanalytic space, it is through this recognition that an analyst and patient can experience themselves on a shared path, and may find a space for human connection in the divided world. I refer to this space as "*the zero*." Only by surrendering ourselves to the nameless universe can human beings move beyond the differences between self and the other, between perpetrator, victim, and bystander.

Chiemi's vignette

Chiemi, an elegant and intelligent female patient in her early sixties, came to see me in an attempt to understand her own life and her emotional conflicts with her mother. At the beginning of our therapeutic work, she expressed a fear of becoming crazy, as her mother had predicted, as well as anger against her mother, who was judgmental and disparaging.

Chiemi was the second child of three. She and her two brothers were born in Nagasaki, like her father, and grew up in Hiroshima, her mother's home. Chiemi said that she had idealized her father, who had passed away several years before she began working with me. For her, her father represented intelligence while her mother was a symbol of anti-intellectualism.

Chiemi's father, a famous professor of natural science, was taciturn and silent at home. Although Chiemi idolized him, she had few recollections of conversations with him. To her, her father was a silent person whose life was consumed by work. He supported many younger students, not only in their academic pursuits but also in their private lives. Chiemi's mother, on the other hand, was not an intellectual. She was a housekeeper whose only pride was in her personal appearance. She was high-maintenance, status-conscious, critical, and discriminatory towards anyone without a prominent academic career or wealthy background. Chiemi remembers her mother judging Chiemi's friends, and even humiliating them on many occasions.

Chiemi and I have worked together for almost ten years on a once a week basis, face to face. We've discussed many issues, including her relational patterns and their profound effects on her social life, her hatred and love for her mother, her expectations for her husband, and for me, and her disappointments in her friends, and me, and so on. Through this analytic process, she came to understand herself and her conflict with her mother, as well as improve her social relations and personal life. About four years into her treatment, she first asked a question that was to come up again and again, "what do people live for in this world?" She told me, "probably this was the real reason why I originally decided to come to see you. This question has been in my mind since childhood, but I was not able to speak of it when I first saw you."

At first, I considered this query to be an expression of her depression, powerlessness, and helplessness. Chiemi often complained about her close friends, saying

"I have always worked for their benefit, but I no longer want to sacrifice myself. Time is precious, and I don't want to lose it for them anymore." I told her that this question indicated her profound disappointment in her relationships and her deep sense of loneliness. She agreed with my understanding, but kept raising the question, "what do people live for?"

During the course of our therapeutic journey, many traumatic events occurred in our community and our own lives. The Great East Japan Earthquake took place in 2011, and my parents in Fukushima were forced to move to another town. At that time, I was in a city far away from them. I did not go to help them immediately after the earthquake, and I criticized myself for being merely a bystander.

A few years later, I began a research project, interviewing survivors of the 9/11 attacks, the Great Hanshin-Awaji Earthquake[2] and the Great East Japan Earthquake. I myself witnessed the 9/11 attacks while living in New York City, but I had refused to address the event. I never spoke about the attacks and never watched television programs about them. I behaved as if it had never happened until I embarked on this research. Soon after I began the project, my father passed away. Since I was forced to skip some of Chiemi's sessions to attend the funeral and related events, she knew that my father had died.

A few years later, Chiemi's mother died after several months of self-sacrificing care by Chiemi. A year after that, her town suffered a pair of natural disasters. Although Chiemi did not lose anything of importance, many friends and colleagues lost houses, cars, and other personal belongings. Some even died. One friend, who lived in the same region as Chiemi, lost her house and her husband—everything. In session, Chiemi related her shock at seeing such a random assignment of life and death, such a thin line between survivor and victim.

One day, Chiemi told me that she remembered, as a child, asking her father to tell her what he thought people lived for—the same question she repeatedly raised in her therapy. Her father, who usually did not express himself so explicitly, said, "People do not live *for* anything. They live for the sake of living. There is no more reason than this." Chiemi said she had not understood what he had meant at the time, but now she felt she did. Then she told me her father's history.

Chiemi's father was a teenager in Nagasaki when his town was struck by the atomic bomb in 1945. He was in the center of the city but, incredibly, was not severely injured. While escaping the damaged area, he was asked by a dying mother to take care of her baby. He carried the infant to a church, where a priest told him to leave the baby and take care of himself, which he did. Chiemi's father had never related this story to anyone, even his family, until the very moment of his death, almost sixty years later. On his deathbed he told his son that he would like to know if the baby lived, and if it had enrolled in a university to study. Although he did not express his regret verbally, this statement implicitly indicates that he had been living with a sense of guilt all through his life.

Chiemi heard the story a day before her father's death, but only now, through her therapeutic work, did she recognize how many areas of his life were organized around this experience: his devotion to his job and his students, his reticence, and his answer to Chiemi's question, "what do people live for in this world?" All emanated from the silence surrounding this episode in his childhood.

Chiemi and I discussed why she finally understood the importance of her father's story. She recognized that we were both player-witnesses of trauma across generations and times. Chiemi was no longer a simple observer of her father's life, but a person organized by, and in turn, organizing her father's life. The natural disasters she had experienced made her feel that human life is organized around contingency, and that anyone could become a victim, victimizer, or bystander. When Chiemi accepted being in such a world, she could finally live in the possibilities of her father's life.

A few sessions later, Chiemi told me a story about her mother, Fumie, who was also a survivor of the atom bomb. Toward the end of the war, almost all the students in Fumie's junior high school in Hiroshima were taken to the center of the city and ordered to help demolish buildings and houses to prevent fires in the wake of air raids. On the day before the bomb was dropped, a friend of Fumie's did not come to school because of a minor cold. Fumie told her teacher the reason for her friend's absence, and the teacher was very upset. He asked her to tell her friend to come to school next day, which she did. Fumie, however, got her period on that day, and her father kept her home. As a result, she witnessed the atomic cloud from her house, and a few days later learned that her friend had died in the blast. Fumie did not talk about this incident for a long time. It was when Chiemi was in her twenties that her mother told her the story.

One day, while they were out shopping, Fumie suddenly stopped and insisted that they take a different route on another street. Chiemi described her mother's face as sickly and pale as she gave vague explanations, saying that there was a person she did not want to see. Later, Chiemi learned that it was the street where Fumie's friend who was killed by the bomb had lived. Now, at last, Chiemi felt that she could make sense of her mother's judging and humiliating of Chiemi's friends. For Fumie, Chiemi's friendships must have reminded her of the guilt she had lived with since her childhood; and keeping Chiemi's friends away from her might have been Fumie's effort to proactively prevent Chiemi from traumatic regret. Chiemi had found another silence in her family.

Being a player-witness

Knowing her parents' experiences with the two atom bomb attacks, Chiemi was able to connect herself to the history of her family and the world. She no longer felt the strong emotional conflict toward her mother that she had experienced before. She felt that she had found the missing pieces, and no longer sensed strange shadows in her family.

What brought about this change? Was it that we had successfully analyzed Chiemi's past? Or that we had successfully reconstructed her life? You could say so, but I believe that our successes are less meaningful in creating this change than our *surrender*. What was required was for us to surrender ourselves to the original point of Chiemi's history, the *zero*.

All Chiemi's family members had been traumatized. Her father lived in a world organized around "a person who was abandoned and a person who abandoned." Her mother lived in a world divided between "survivor and killed." It took all their energy throughout their lives to maintain silence about these divisions, yet still the traumatization was passed on to the next generation, a phenomenon described by Frie (2017a). Their daughter did not know what human beings live for, but when she herself became a player-witness of trauma and the world's contingency, the divided worlds that had been trans-generated through her parents began to speak to each other. She was no longer a bystander or observer of her parents' lives because she recognized how she *could have been them* if she had been born in their time.

This change in Chiemi's perspective might not have occurred without my own experience of 9/11, the Great East Japan Earthquake, and my father's death. Without these experiences, I would have been merely an observer analyzing my patient's narratives, but through them I was also a player-witness of the traumatic world, a world in which all human beings are connected. Born in a different time, I could have been an a-bomb survivor, like the little girl in the photo of Hiroshima, who looked into the lens of the camera with empty eyes; Chiemi could have been a survivor of the Great East Japan Earthquake; her mother could have been killed by an a-bomb and her father also killed, together with the infant in his arms. No one knows how they might have lived or died in a different context, but everyone knows that there are alternate possibilities in their lives. At the point of *zero*, we can say that there are infinite possibilities, and that it is the only point in which all people can be connected to each other.

Notes

1 The Great East Japan Earthquake struck the eastern half of Japan on March 11, 2011, and triggered a huge tsunami, which destroyed some of the emergency generating systems of the nuclear power plant located along the coast of Fukushima. From the 12th to the 15th of March, the plant underwent three nuclear meltdowns, hydrogen-air explosions, and the release of a great deal of radioactive material. By September 10, 2019, 15,898 people lost their lives, 2,531 people were missing, and 6,157 people were injured from the earthquake and tsunami (Emergency Disaster Countermeasures Headquarters of the National Police Agency, 2019). By November, 2019, in Fukushima Prefecture alone, 4,109 people had lost their lives, one person was missing, 183 people were injured, and 41,916 people were still evacuated due to the accident in the nuclear plant (Disaster Prevention Headquarter of Fukushima Prefecture, 2019).

2 The Great Hanshin Earthquake occurred on January 17, 1995, in Hyogo Prefecture, Japan. It measured 7.3 on the Richter scale. By May 19, 2006, 6,434 people lost their lives, three people were missing, and 40,092 people were injured (The Great Hanshin-Awaji Earthquake Memorial Disaster Reduction and Human Renovation Institution, 2016).

PART II

Human suffering and the experience of being human

6

BEING THROWN INTO THE WORLD WITHOUT INFORMED CONSENT

A patient who is a survivor of the Great East Japan Earthquake described her experience of that event to me, saying, "I was exposed to the massive disaster suddenly, without advance notice. I felt completely powerless." Another patient, a survivor of serious physical abuse by his parents, angrily told me, "I did not choose them as my parents. I did not grant them permission to give birth to me."

For both these patients, their subjective experience is affected by a traumatic event that strikes them without their knowledge and willing agreement or permission. In other words, informed consent is missing at a crucial moment in their lives.

It is beyond people's knowledge when, how, and in what way a natural disaster, accident, war, or life-threatening disease may strike them. They cannot know in advance the degree of damage or the intensity and duration of the lasting effects of these events. They have no space in which to make an autonomous decision about whether or not to accept the event, and no way to give consent.

Similarly, when people become stuck in an abusive relationship, their agency is coerced, lost to deception or both. Even if a person feels that they have acknowledged the risks or effects of the harmful relationship and consented to it, the normal process of autonomous decision-making may be distorted or constrained. If a father sexually abuses his daughter and the daughter grants him permission, it does not mean that she adequately knows the meaning and risks of a sexual relationship with her father. Ferenczi's (1949) concept, "confusion of the tongues" is a good example of coercion and deception in the failure of informed consent.

But the inability to give consent when experiencing an unexpected event does not always traumatize people. We are exposed to most events without consent, and only rarely are we knowledgeable about the content, characteristic features, potential influence, or risks of an event in advance. Walking down the street on a rainy day, a car splashes muddy water on you, or a friend calls to cancel on the day of an appointment so that she can go out with her boyfriend; as a rule, such events do not traumatize people. Indeed, as Loewald (1979) describes, we "experience ourselves as agents, notwithstanding the fact that we were born without our informed consent and did not pick our parents" (p.761).

So, in what cases *would* people be traumatized, or not, by being exposed to an event without consent?

This chapter begins with a review of the general discussion on informed consent in medical ethics and explores its specific application to psychoanalysis. I also discuss the impossibility of giving informed consent to traumatic events. I then review the self-psychological and intersubjective literature that explores trauma from the perspective of the "psychology of being human" (Togashi, 2014c; Togashi & Kottler, 2015).

The discussion of informed consent and traumatic events is related to the existential anguish of living in our contemporary world, a world that is increasingly experienced as uncertain. This relationship is explored via the case vignette of a patient who suffers from complex trauma; a history in which she was neither informed about or able to consent to various events in her life. Finally, I discuss how the lack of informed consent to a traumatic event can violate one's sense of responsibility, and how we may undertake the process of *granting informed consent retrospectively*.

Experience without informed consent

Informed consent is an ethical concept commonly used in medical practice and research, and refers to a person, voluntarily and with foreknowledge, authorizing another's intrusive actions on their persons. It is an issue of subjective experience in the sense that it prioritizes autonomy or self-ownership as a basic human right (Archard, 2008; Pateman, 2002); it is a relational issue in the sense that one person is obligated to disclose a necessary set of information, and another person must authorize the action (Beauchamp & Childress, 1994; Amer, 2013). Beauchamp and Childress (1994) give an outline of the elements of informed consent as follows:

(I) Threshold Elements (Preconditions)

1. Competence (to understand and decide)
2. Voluntariness (in deciding)

(II) Information Elements

1. Disclosure (of material information)
2. Recommendation (of plan)
3. Understanding (of 3 and 4)

(III) Consent Elements

1. Decision (in favor of a plan)
2. Authorization (of chosen plan)

(Beauchamp and Childress, 1994, pp.145–146)

Many philosophers and theorists in medical ethics have struggled to find the essential value of informed consent, and in what sense the failure of informed consent is wrong (President's Commission for the Study of Ethical Problems in Medicine and Biomedical and Behavioral Research, 1982; Beauchamp and Childress, 2001; Pateman, 2002; O'Neill, 2002; Deutscher Bundestag, 2004; Archard, 2008; Amer, 2013). Some emphasize a fundamental interest in autonomy, an individual's freedom from external coercion and social interference in the crucial issues of his or her life; others emphasize a person's radical independence in leading his or her life. Despite some differences of emphasis, these thinkers all advance the view that the ethical foundation of informed consent is based on respect for self-determination.

Archard (2008) emphasizes self-ownership as a fundamental ethical principle, separate from and in addition to autonomy. He uses the example of a non-consensual mouth swab, an act which is neither harmful nor invasive to the person's body, but which is generally considered to be wrongful. He thinks that the violation of autonomy does not fully explain the fundamental ethical wrong in this case, for the value of autonomy is, for him, found in making decisions about *crucial* issues in a person's life, and the mouth swab is not intrusive or painful enough to be seen as a critical life decision. Furthermore, if the usurpation of autonomy is the basic wrong, a mouth swab taken when a person is sleeping, without awareness, can be justified. Archard (2008) contends that the basic and distinctive wrong in this case can be seen in the violation of self-ownership of the body.

What is common to these discussions is the observation that informed consent is a reification of a basic human right and relates to ways in which a person is treated by the other as being human. In one's subjective experience, a person believes that she is at the center of self-determination and self-ownership. When that belief is violated, namely when a person experiences a failure of informed consent, she may be disappointed in herself, and may be unable to experience herself as being human. Thus, informed consent is not only an ethical issue in medical practice and research, but also an experiential issue in human life.

Every day and at every moment, human beings are subject to *reality without consent* in events both trivial and critical. Even when a person undergoes a medical procedure *with* informed consent, it is not fully consensual in relation to a complete life experience, because he or she has not given consent or authorization to the event which resulted in the need for surgery.

Imagine a person who faces the loss of a loved one in a massive earthquake. There are no preconditions that will make him competent to understand and voluntarily decide to accept the earthquake. No one could have disclosed detailed information about the personal impact of the earthquake in advance, nor has anyone given him recommendations for a future plan for his life. He is not in a position to make a decision or authorize a chosen plan.

Another example is child abuse. Envision a child who has been abused by her mother. Again, the preconditions cannot be met; the child is not competent enough to understand the real reasons for the abuse, not able to understand that her mother's uncontrolled irritation is caused by events unrelated to herself. The child's commitment to her mother is not voluntarily decided. No information about an abusive relationship is disclosed, and the "recommendation of plan" is inadequate and often coercive or deceptive. The child's "decision" and authorization of the chosen plan is not voluntary in any authentic manner.

Clearly, most human experiences are given without informed consent. So how does one maintain a sense of being human in this world? If we recognize the radical failure of informed consent, in what sense is informed consent meaningful for a human life?

Trauma and the psychology of being human

A review of recent studies of trauma, in self psychology and intersubjective-systems theory, from the perspective of the "psychology of being human" (Togashi, 2014c, 2014d, 2014e; Togashi & Kottler, 2015; Jacobs, 2017) indicates that living in this world is inherently traumatic and antithetical to the elements of informed consent.

The "psychology of being human" refers to a shift of emphasis, in theory and clinical practice, from how a human being experiences himself as cohesive to how a human being experiences himself as *being human*. From this perspective, human anguish, which often traumatizes people, is understood as an outgrowth of seeking ways to be authentically human while facing the impermanence and contingency of the world, and the radical alterity of the other. The "psychology of being human" includes what some analysts refer to as the "ethical turn in psychoanalysis" (Baraitser, 2008; Corpt, 2016; Brothers, 2014; Orange, 2013, 2014a, 2014b; Sucharov, 2014; Weisel-Barth, 2015).

In the psychology of being human, trauma has been discussed from two different angles: existential trauma, which is embedded into a person's anguish of being in the unknowable, unpredictable, and contingent world; and relational trauma, which is rooted in a person's struggle to accommodate him or herself to a relationship while maintaining a sense of agency. The classifications are not necessarily linked with event types, but in general, existential trauma is most often seen in our experience of natural disasters or social turmoil such as war, industrial accidents, terrorism, and crimes. Relational trauma is related to abuses, domestic violence, or bullying. The two are frequently intermixed, and the experience of a single event often has both faces.

Existential Trauma

Researchers who study existential trauma explore the subjective meaning, for patients, of living in an uncontrollable, unpredictable, and unknowable world with existential vulnerability (Stolorow, 2007; Brothers, 2008; Togashi, 2014a, 2014b). For these writers, trauma is not a pathology to be cured or fixed, but a way of living in this world, and the aim of psychoanalysis is to find a way of living while facing a sense of uncertainty.

Stolorow (2007) contends that trauma shatters "the absolutisms of everyday life" (Stolorow, 2007, p.16); the illusory belief system through which an individual views the world as stable and predictable. Trauma, in his view, disturbs the survivor's experience of temporality: "experiences of trauma become freeze-framed into an eternal present in which one remains forever trapped" (2007, p. 20).

The experience of trauma confronts individuals with their existential vulnerability, human limitation, finiteness, and impermanence. For Stolorow, trauma is an experience of context-embedded unbearable emotional pain, which can be integrated only by being understood by the other who knows "the darkness of our common finiteness." (Stolorow, 2010, p.35).

Brothers (2008) argues that trauma plunges our relational systems into chaos and exposes us to experiences of unbearable uncertainty about our psychological survival. She views traumatic experiences as complex phenomena that involve the destruction of certainty about one's sense of "going-on-being" (Winnicott, 1956) as well as strenuous efforts to regain that sense. These efforts often take the form of reducing the complexity of lived experience by the creation of rigid dualities that dominate the victim's relational world. Because analysts are no more strangers to trauma than their patients, these patterns often come to organize therapeutic relationships.

In a brief essay (Togashi, 2010), I discussed the Japanese esthetic "Mono-no-aware," a concept involving the belief and acceptance that change is a constant and that there are no absolutes in the human world. An individual embracing this philosophy is motivated to work through the anguish associated with the conditions of finitude and impermanence. For such a person, human tragedy comes from contingency in the world (Togashi, 2014a, 2014b). This concept can be applied to the therapeutic domain, where it is important in the psychoanalysis of traumatized patients for analyst and patient to share the sense of "no absolutes" and the irrationality of living in this world.

Atwood (2011) contends that *all* trauma can be called "epistemological trauma." In a fictional dialogue between a psychiatrist, Dr. E and himself, he writes:

> An epistemological trauma is an event that undercuts someone's faith in what previously had been believed to be true. It is an event or situation in a person's life that contradicts what had been a matter of the given theretofore. The effect of such a trauma is the shattering of confidence in one's own mind. Such a collapse of trust in oneself can lead to terrible things, even, in the extreme, to an experience of personal annihilation. It makes a person feel he or she doesn't know anything anymore, and nothing can make it better.
>
> *(Atwood, 2011, p.396)*

These studies suggest that existential trauma is a subjectively experienced condition of this world. People cannot obtain foreknowledge about the world they live in, and they cannot meaningfully supply consent to their fate. They are confronted with evidence that they themselves are ultimately incapable of determining the direction of their own lives; their belief in self-determination is always at risk. The only environment in which people can possibly experience their lives as self-determined may be in an interpersonal field, or "relational home" (Stolorow, 2007, 2008), but this, too, may not be experienced as sure and certain.

Relational trauma

In contemporary self psychology and intersubjective-systems theory, relational trauma has mainly been discussed as a person's struggle to balance accommodation to an interpersonal environment with maintaining a sense of personal agency, and being him or herself in relationship to other human beings. This type of trauma is organized around coercion and deception. Even if a certain type of agreement is made between a person and the other, consent is not obtained based on full knowledge of the conditions.

Brandchaft (2001; see also Brandchaft, Doctors, & Sorter, 2010) discusses an intersubjective process in which a child assimilates herself to the wishes of the parents. The child's authentic self is vulnerable in this case; the parents cannot act sufficiently in concert with the child. Brandchaft emphasizes that the child, afraid of the destructive loss of emotional connection, is compelled to maintain the relationship, and may lose the space for reflection on her experience of self and relationship. This type of intersubjective process, which he refers to as "pathological accommodation," is, in a certain sense, a relationship without consent—or more precisely, a relationship which is *not ready* for informed consent.

Stern (2009), discussing the self psychological concept of empathy from a contemporary relational, and intersubjective perspective, sees the traumatized patient as feeling "too alone, yet, paradoxically, too much at the mercy of the Other from whom she does not feel entirely differentiated, simply to 'be with' her own feelings, recognized ('mentalized') as such" (p.143). For Stern, relational trauma is the loss of the optimal balance of closeness and distance in the relationship, a loss in which the otherness of the other cannot be sufficiently experienced and the sufferer's subjectivity can no longer be optimally recognized. In this situation, he says, the only way a person survives is to stay within the relationship, albeit with some enactment or externalization of the sense of imprisonment.

My discussion of the development and failure of a twinship experience, from a dynamic systems view, also indicates that relational trauma is a failure to maintain the optimal balance of similarity and difference between a person and the other (Togashi, 2012; Togashi & Kottler, 2012b). A traumatized person is often afraid of finding himself in the other and vice versa. Finding similarity in each other, in this context, is often experienced as losing the uniqueness of being.

The essential aspect of relational trauma, in these discussions, is not necessarily the violation of the sense of self-determination, for people often do not recognize that they have been coerced, or are not conscious of being deceived. They may experience themselves as being self-determined and yet be deeply injured by the relationship, as in the daughter-father relationship referred to at the beginning of this chapter as an example of Ferenczi's "confusion of the tongues" (Ferenczi, 1949). A daughter may experience herself as self-determined and as choosing the relationship on her own, when in fact the decision is made under circumstances of coercion and deception.

In relational trauma the issue is the violation of the *belief* in self-ownership. Traumatized individuals are confronted with evidence that they are ultimately incapable of owning their minds and bodies. The intersubjective field they are embedded in is also not their own. Even if they are satisfied with a certain amount of intimacy with others, the basic sense of self-ownership can be lost, and they will not experience themselves as the owners of their own lives.

What we now have to consider is whether or not the violation of the belief in self-determination and self-ownership is the basic wrong of existential/relational trauma. If the lack of self-determination and self-ownership is simply how this world is, then trauma does not destroy a basic human right but reveals the very impossibility of self-determination and self-ownership, and we can no longer consider these to be the essential values of informed consent. We must redefine these values for a human being who lives in this existential anguish.

Case vignette

A female Japanese patient, Mizuho, in her thirties, came to see me for psychoanalytic psychotherapy complaining of suicidal ideation, self-cutting, eating disorder, and sexual promiscuity. She was highly intelligent, had graduated from a master's program at a prominent university, and worked in a highly responsible position.

Since her childhood, Mizuho had had a sexual relationship with her cousin, who was four years older than her and lived in the same household, raised by Mizuho's parents. In the year before Mizuho came to see me, the cousin killed himself by hanging. Mizuho's symptoms began soon after, and she had to quit her job. Although Mizuho and I worked together twice a week face-to-face, we often needed an extra session because she occasionally suffered from memory loss and because she had a strong wish to kill herself. Her therapy lasted for seven years.

In my initial work with Mizuho, I was overwhelmed by my powerlessness to deal with the reality she faced. Mizuho's father, also a sophisticated professional, was often hospitalized for bipolar disorder. He was violent with all members of his family; Mizuho described episodes where he destroyed a TV set and smashed windows in their home with a metal baseball bat. Mizuho's mother did not do anything to protect her children and often escaped from their home temporarily, leaving them behind.

It is no wonder that Mizuho and her cousin, seeking a way of surviving in such a harsh world, came to be sexually connected with each other, even though the relationship led to further suffering and anguish. When the cousin, who was the center of Mizuho's suffering and love, hung himself, it was she who discovered his dead body and took it down. She related this to me without emotion, "I don't know how I was able to lower him to the floor by myself. His body lost all muscle tension and was extraordinarily heavy."

In session, Mizuho did not show any changes of facial expression or tone of voice. The only signs of emotion she displayed were slight tears that appeared regardless of context. I looked for a way to access her emotional experience and encouraged her to voice her feelings but, not surprisingly, her emotions went unexpressed. Instead, she reacted to my encouragement by cutting herself or indicating suicidal ideation.

For the first four and a half years of psychotherapy, I constantly feared that Mizuho would kill herself. She had lost her cousin to suicide, and she continued to live in the room in which he had killed himself. She said, "When I look at the door header [where my cousin hung himself], I feel myself getting sucked into it." Nevertheless, she was unable to move to another room, because it was the only place where she experienced herself as being alive.

I did what I could to protect Mizuho: I kept contact with her psychiatrist and talked to her mother. I set up an emergency network for hospitalization in case of a suicide attempt on her part, and asked her to give me a rope she had acquired for that purpose in order to keep it until her suicidal ideation settled. She told me that she was not able to promise not to kill herself, but she did, finally, make a commitment to call me or her psychiatrist if she felt the urge to kill herself. Whenever she came to her sessions, I checked to see how severe the ideation was. She was hospitalized four times during her seven-year psychotherapy.

I recognized that if Mizuho made up her mind to kill herself, I could not stop her. Even after doing everything I could, there was no way of controlling her mind. I recognized that there was a part of her which I never reached or understood, *because she was not me*, but the other. I was chilled by this undeniable fact.

While Mizuho was largely impassive in sessions, I saw something in her face that made me feel I had to respond. She said that she was afraid of becoming a burden to me. She did not feel that she deserved to be in my office, and occasionally suggested that she should leave analysis without expressing any particular reasons other than a sense of invalidity or inadequacy. I myself was confused. Since I made it a principle never to see more than one patient who demanded from me the time and energy that Mizuho did, I kept checking myself to see if I was capable of treating her. I oscillated between feelings that I could and could not do so.

Finally, I had the idea that Mizuho should send me an email at a fixed time, 10 pm each night, to confirm that she was alive. It was my responsibility to protect her and it was her responsibility to reassure me, because I was fearful about treating her in this uncontrollable situation. We discussed this many times before we imposed this method, and agreed that I would not reply to her message unless she showed clearly her wish for me to do so. We did this every day for three years. I did not feel this process as a burden. Her condition was so serious that it was natural for us to do it. It was nothing less than a way to protect her life; she did not have any expectations other than that, and I did not either.

We did not expect that we could easily understand each other. Indeed, she said, "I do not think that you can understand me. I loved my cousin who I thought of as my brother and I had slept with. Then, I cared for his dead body. I had been repeatedly assaulted by my father and many times feared being killed by him. There is no expectation in me to be understood. No way."

In regard to her cousin, Mizuho said, "I did not think we understood each other, either. I think that we were simply connected with each other."

What Mizuho and I recognized was that she was not able to do anything to consent to her own life. Like any other person, she was not able to choose in what condition, between whom, and in what way she was born. She did not know that her cousin wanted to kill himself, and she was not in a position to withhold authorization for him to act it out. The only exception to her feeling of a lack of consent was her feeling about her mother, who had often escaped from their violent home. Mizuho said, "I know that she could not do anything in such an environment. I understand and can accept her behavior." Mizuho said that she was disappointed in her mother, who told her many times, "I am so sorry. I cannot do anything," but she was able to consent to it.

Approximately five years after Mizuho's therapy began, our main theme became her sexual promiscuity. I had been unable to raise this topic actively for the first three or four years because I was afraid for her survival. But around this time, I felt I could pick up on it. I felt it was unacceptable that she did not say anything, either in advance or in retrospect, about seeking out one-night stands. I recognized that such acting-out was still necessary for her, and I did not want her to stop doing it immediately, but I felt increasingly uncomfortable about her not being able to share important information about her condition.

I finally asked her, "Please let me know when you have made up your mind to have sex with someone you don't know. Your sexual behavior looks risky. I do not ask because I want you to stop, but because I want to know what happens to you. Give me a chance to know your life because it affects me. I need informed consent." Mizuho opened her eyes wide and said with surprise, "Do you really want to know about this? It is a new experience for me." She had thought that I might have not been interested in her life. After a while, she gradually stopped her promiscuous behavior.

Toward the end of her therapy, we discussed many times how we had met and how we had been together for seven years. She told me that at the beginning she felt uncertain about me and what I could do for her; I told her that I felt uncertain about her and what she wanted from me. We both knew that our encounter was meaningful, and we both felt that having been responsible for each other was valid. She now felt that she deserved to be in session with me, saying, "I agree to go on living."

Our work in session was not intended to get rid of the trauma or to fix her life, but rather to give meaning to each experience in order to find a way to live in the world. It was a way for her to recognize the impossibility of self-ownership and self-determination, while at the same time understanding and authorizing her own life in her subjective experience. Our work was a process by which she experienced herself being validated to be in the world. She ultimately enrolled in a doctoral program and became a researcher.

Discussion and conclusion

Mizuho was a survivor on a fierce battlefield, subject to various kinds of violence. At her core, as an organizing principle, there was an overwhelming powerlessness and helplessness. She was not able to understand what people did to her, nor to accept, authorize, or reject it. The world, for her, was experienced as unknowable, uncertain, impermanent, and unpredictable. The only thing of which she felt certain was that nobody wanted to understand or access her experience.

Failure of informed consent in Mizuho's life

Mizuho's traumatization was complex and encompassed many areas. She was born into a violent family and was exposed to her father's physical abuse for many years. As she herself said, she did not wish to be born in that environment, but was thrown into the family as a child, without consent.

In this environment, Mizuho became sexually connected to her cousin. In a sense, the relationship offered her hope. She was able to have a love object. She probably originally experienced their relationship as certain and peaceful. She felt she was informed, and was confident in what her cousin wanted of her and she wanted from him. They were in agreement, although they did not know what the relationship actually meant. Faced with her cousin's suicide, however, Mizuho had to recognize that her confidence in their relationship was illusory, and her cousin contained a radical alterity that she was never able to access. Her relationship with him, which had been a source of hope for a peaceful refuge, became a source of traumatization.

Looking at Mizuho's experience in terms of informed consent, we can say that she was not competent to understand and voluntarily decide about events in her life. She was not informed—in advance or in retrospect—about the meaning of why she had to be born into this family, why she was abused by her father, or why she needed the sexual relationship with her cousin. She was not in a position to make a decision in favor of a "plan" or authorize a chosen "plan." Her clock was frozen in a traumatized present.

Mizuho's relationship with her mother seemed to have a different quality. She was wounded by witnessing her mother escaping her father's violence and temporarily leaving Mizuho and her cousin behind. But Mizuho told me that it was not a big deal to her, and she could not blame her mother for this. She said, "I know that she could not help herself in such an environment." Mizuho acknowledged and accepted her mother's behavior and was able to retrospectively authorize her escape, despite the fact that it was not based in mutual agreement. She was disappointed in her mother, who many times told her, "I am so sorry. I cannot do anything," but felt that she understood her. In other words, retrospective informed consent was a significant factor in Mizuho's experience, although we do not know whether the experience was less traumatic because of her retrospective informed consent, or if she was able to consent to her mother's behavior because she was less traumatized by it. And, of course, the source of the trauma still remains, namely the lack of mutual agreement about her mother's escape.

Informed consent in a therapeutic process

A major aspect of my psychotherapeutic work with Mizuho was that there always remained an anonymous part in the relationship. She had that in her subjectivity which I felt to be inaccessible, and she also felt that there was a part of my subjectivity which she could not reach. There was an intersubjective conjunction that was out of sight of both of us, but made us feel connected and responsible for understanding each other.

Mizuho was emotionless and wordless at the beginning of our work. Even in response to simple queries, she spoke only a few ambiguous words, and I felt it was hard to understand her. In addition to this, the risk of her suicide was enough to make me to abandon the illusion that we could easily be empathic with each other. Even toward the end of her therapy, she chose not to tell me about her sexual promiscuity in detail. In a certain sense, I experienced a lack of informed consent. Because of this inaccessibility, we were deeply motivated to become knowledgeable about and confident in each other, while still recognizing the unknowability in our relationship.

In this environment, all I could do as a therapist was to discuss and talk with her, without interpretation. A good example is the process by which we came to agreement about her regular email messages. For a few months after the idea came into my mind, I thought about the transference-countertransference meaning and potential merit and risk of the idea. I finally decided to ask her how she felt about it. She nodded at the idea, but I was not certain what the nod meant because her expression was typically unclear, and she tended to almost automatically assimilate herself to the other. I could not analyze or interpret her nodding because interpretation was meaningless in a context where she herself was not certain about her own mind. Yet I did talk about, explain, discuss, and regulate the idea; and she talked about, explained, and discussed how she felt. When she and I finally authorized the plan, it was, indeed, a process of mutual informed consent.

I maintain that informed consent is not a condition but an ongoing process in a dyadic relationship. Ultimately, informed consent cannot be achieved in a human relationship but is instead a dialogue through which people negotiate, discuss, talk, and attempt to understand each other when they happen to meet.

When Mizuho chose to be hospitalized, we did not have an opportunity to discuss her actions beforehand, because it was always in the midst of an emergency. In other words, I did not have a chance to consent to her hospitalization. In each case, she herself decided to be hospitalized without letting me participate in her decision-making. Her psychological condition was too severe for her to explain why she felt it necessary to be hospitalized. However, after she left the hospital, we talked about the decision process and came to a place of mutual consent. I told her, frankly, that I often felt fearful because I was uncertain about her condition and thought. This discussion was not an effort to analyze or interpret her behavior, but an attempt to make sense of what happened together (Orange, 1995). The essential meaning of informed consent in a therapeutic process is to provide this sense of responsibility.

When I asked Mizuho to tell me about her sexual activity in advance, she had an interesting reaction. She was surprised when I told her, "I like to know what happens in your life because it affects me." She thought that I would not be interested in her life, and she did not know that her behavior could affect me. Over time, we came to feel responsible for talking about our feelings and thoughts with each other. This sense of responsibility for mutual talking, sharing, discussing, and agreeing changed our work.

Mizuho told me that she was never asked to talk about herself, even by her cousin. Before her cousin killed himself, she dated several boys without telling him. She was not trying to keep this a secret from him, and she believed that she would have told him if he had asked her. She did not feel that not telling him would injure him, and she did not feel guilty because she did not believe that her behavior or her being had any influence on others. She did not have to explain herself to anyone. In her relationship with her cousin, there was no sense of responsibility for informed consent about each other's behavior. After our discussion, she came to the painful recognition that her dating another boy without telling her cousin might have bothered him and may have contributed to his decision to kill himself.

Clinical implications

In this chapter, informed consent is defined, in a broad sense, not only as an ethical issue or treatment process in professional work but also as a way of committing to the human world and human interaction. A traumatized patient is faced with uncontrollability, unknowability, and unpredictability in the human world and with coercion, deception, or pathological accommodation in human relationships. Some face both types of trauma. In all cases, the patient experiences the violation of belief in self-determination, the violation of belief in self-ownership of mind, or both.

But what we have found is that the distinctive wrong in a failure of informed consent in the intersubjective process is neither the violation of self-determination or self-ownership, but the violation of a sense of responsibility. Self-determination and self-ownership are usually experienced as basic human rights, and, I believe, adequately describe values in intrapsychic processes of the mind.

However, looking at our case vignette from the intersubjective perspective, the failure of informed consent led to Mizuho's feeling that she did not have the basic right to participate in the intersubjective process and did not deserve to be in "a connection with a brother or a sister who knows the same darkness" (Stolorow, 2007, p.49). Informed consent in the intersubjective process calls on the idea that human beings are responsible for each other; that each of us is responsible for being a human being among other human beings (Kohut, 1984).

Mizuho's case suggests that efforts to obtain mutual informed consent to the therapeutic process need not necessarily be undertaken in advance. The efforts of patient and analyst to obtain informed consent in retrospect can make the patient's experience less traumatic and lead to a sense of responsibility. In this process, both participants are responsible for talking, understanding, listening, and agreeing with each other; it proceeds along with the process of recognizing the unknowable, as well as the connected, aspects in their intersubjective field. Through this process, a patient comes to consent to the attitude of the world and the other, while being informed that he or she is being human.

As Loewald (1979) says, human beings are born without informed consent. However, even after we are born, we can subjectively consent to our fate and authorize our own lives. This perspective is also consistent with my recent study of being human (Togashi, 2014c; Chapter 8); it is a basic element of a sense of being human that a person shares with the other (in many cases, a parent), how they have been born, and how they have been together. A human birth given without informed consent will be humanized by the mutual process of retrospective informed consent.

Creating a space for responsibility[1]

As we have seen, informed consent is organized around the reflection of human dignity, irreplaceability, and taking responsibility. What does "taking responsibility" mean in a psychoanalytic relationship—not as a technical issue but an ethical one?

In the history of psychoanalysis, until the emergence of the "ethical turn," the issue of responsibility had been mainly discussed from two perspectives: etiological and technical. From the etiological perspective, the discussion focused on whether or not a patient (or an analyst) is responsible for his or her own pathology, unconscious wishes, and fantasies (Freud, 1925a; Klein, 1976; Schwartz, 1984; Meissner, 2003). From the perspective of psychoanalytic technique, the emphasis is on whether or not, or in what way, an analyst should attribute a problem that emerges in a therapeutic field to his own failure to understand or respond to his patient's need (Grotstein, 1999; Preston & Shumsky, 2004). The ethical turn goes beyond such traditional discussions and looks at an analyst's ability to respond to the patient's call as a human being. To some degree, an analyst serves the demands of his patient before, or beyond, being aware of himself in his professional role, and devotes himself to a relationship with or to his patient, as discussed in Chapter 3.

Informed consent, from this perspective, is born at the moment of an analyst's responding to her patient's demand, prior to the awareness of her professional role. Reflection on informed consent shows us that a human being spends her life taking on responsibility, not only for her own life, that she has never chosen, but also for the past pains and sufferings, the present feelings and anguish, and the future wishes and hopes of the others she meets. When a person sees someone collapse on the street, they reach out to help. There is no informed consent in a technical sense, but there is, in that moment, the birth of human relationship. A person responds to the call of the Other and both participants can find themselves in the fallen person's demand; the consent they make at the very moment will create not only the present relationship but a future commitment. Similarly, in a therapeutic relationship an analyst helps her patient; the mere fact that the suffering patient is there is sufficient reason for taking on this responsibility.

Baraitser (2008) describes this type of responsibility beautifully. She states:

> First and foremost there is the Other. Subjectivity is seen to emerge through a relation to this radical alterity, or otherness. I argue that, in fact, the maternal could be seen as both an emblematic and enigmatic formation of this subjectivity "called into being" through the relation to an "other" who, in this case, is a child. I contend that an interrupting, tantruming, crying, demanding, changing, questioning, loving, unpredictable, and ultimately unknowable other that is a child is a particular kind of other, the response to whom calls us, as maternal subjects, into being.
>
> *(Baraitser, 2008, p.90)*

Baraitser maintains that this is a good example of Levinasian ethics; a caregiver's ability to respond to the call for responsibility from the Other even before being aware of his own existence. I would say that this is the very moment of birth of informed consent in human relationships.

An analyst responds to the patient's call for responsibility and discovers herself on demands from the patient, demands that she has never chosen. The analyst takes responsibility for statements about the patient's past, current, and future life, a life which she herself can neither predict nor control.

Orange (2017) describes the ethical interplay between a patient's demand and an analyst's response beautifully. First, she states, "our patients entrust their very souls to our care, not knowing if they will emerge healed or further wounded. There is no real informed consent for the work we do" (Orange, 2017, p.36). Then, "the face of the suffering other (Orange, 2011) creates a demand on this analyst to stand by his patient without much investment in results" (Orange, 2017, p.38). Through this process, the patient has "his steadfast affirmation of her human dignity and worth no matter what constituted his fragile informed consent to the ethical situation into which he had been thrown" (Orange, 2017, p.38).

Here I would like to expand this discussion to include a mutually recognizing system of taking responsibility in a psychoanalytic setting. There is no question that

Mizuho's case indicates that she created a demand on me to stand by her, even without being invested in results. It is also important to note that a suffering therapist creates a demand on the patient to stand by the therapist. Mizuho knew that she herself could not control her strong suicidal ideations and wishes; her therapist was frightened by them and suffered from her fragile informed consent to working together. It was in this context that her therapist came up with the idea of her sending a regular email message to him every day, which was the only way he could see for him to stand by her and take on the responsibility for her suffering. It was also true that this was the only way he (and also she) could see for Mizuho to stand by her analyst in this situation, and to take on responsibility for *his* suffering.

The psychoanalytic relationship is not symmetric (Teicholz, 1998; Aron, 1999; Baraitser, 2008). An analyst is responsible for his patient's mental health, while a patient cannot be required to take responsibility for her analyst's. If an analyst asks his patient to do so, it may be seen as an exploitation. Once we see the psychoanalytic relationship as being organized by two human beings, however, we see that it is no wonder that a patient spontaneously comes to respond to the analyst's call if she sees the suffering in her therapist's face. The patient responds as a human being, without thinking of her role as a patient. In this situation, the patient's behavior should be distinguished from a manifestation of masochism or submission. As British object relational analyst Ian Suttie (1935) beautifully describes, a child anguishes over not only the circumstance in which her caregivers do not love her, but also the circumstance in which her love for her parents is not accepted by them.

If a patient is given an opportunity to take responsibility for her therapist's suffering, how can she take advantage of it? Responsibility for the Other lies in the creation of a space for letting the Other take responsibility for her. I, as Mizuho's therapist, took responsibility for her by creating a space in which she could take responsibility for me, by creating my own space. The only difference was that the first step for mutual responsibility was mine. It is part of the fundamental ethics of our professional work to create a space for mutual responsibility, for the future therapeutic relationship, in the present relationship—a way of making the impossibility of informed consent possible in an intersubjective field.

Note

1 This section was originally written as a reply (Togashi, 2017b) to Dr. Donna Orange's (2017) rich commentary to my article, the original version of this chapter. I would like to express my gratitude to her for her thoughtful and beautiful discussion, which sheds fresh light on my work and highlights some significant points that I myself did not recognize. Her poignant discussion articulates my thinking in clear and definitive terms.

7

FROM TRAUMATIZED INDIVIDUALITY TO BEING HUMAN WITH OTHERS

Intersubjective taboo and unspoken reality

Traumatized patients often experience themselves as being alienated from human society. While they strongly desire connectedness with others who have suffered similar anguish, they are simultaneously afraid of accepting the possibility that anyone could understand their suffering, and avoid environments in which they might share their experience. An essential aspect of their traumatization is that they cannot feel their experience as accessible to anyone else.

A good example is Hideki, a patient discussed by Togashi and Kottler (2012b, 2015). As a child, Hideki had been physically and psychologically abused by his mother. Before seeking individual therapy, he participated in a group process for survivors of parental abuse. He found that, although he was willing to listen to group members' histories, he could not tolerate them claiming that their experiences had been similar to his. He felt these members' accounts as intrusions into his own special place, and worried that they might steal the significance of an experience that had been the core of his being from childhood.

Traumatized patients like Hideki often avoid recognizing the apparent similarities between their experiences and those of others, insisting that their experiences are different and unique. This uniqueness becomes an aspect of pain and pride in their traumatization, and they rely on it, even at the cost of being alienated from others. In other words, they withdraw into their painful pride, into a *traumatized individuality*.

For traumatized patients like Hideki, the effort to find "a brother or sister who knows the same darkness" (Stolorow, 2007, p.49) is preordained to fail. Such patients need a relational home in which they can experience themselves as being human. Seeing themselves as unique human beings, however, means rejecting being with others and being with others means being unable to see themselves as unique human beings. How can a therapist find a way of working through this dilemma to develop a dyadic process that might transform traumatized individuality into a sense of being human with others?

Sense of individuality

Individuality, in this discussion, does not refer to the state of being a person, or to a developmental achievement in object relationship such as separation-individuation, but refers to the state or quality of one's being which is recognized as differentiated from another. The *sense of individuality* is the subjective experience of oneself as a human being who is absolutely differentiated from others. It is organized around the uniqueness of one's being, as opposed to generality, and can often become the core of one's sense of self.

It is no wonder that a traumatic experience is often used by a patient as part of a sense of individuality. A traumatic event attacks a person discretely, unexpectedly, and fortuitously. Although an event may impact a whole population, the subjective meaning of it is discrete and different for each person. There are no two identical traumatic experiences; a traumatic experience is always personal and unique.

A survivor of the Great East Japan Earthquake lost one of his family members to the tsunami and was then forced to evacuate his home and move to another town due to radiation emissions from the nuclear accident. He felt that his pain and suffering could not be understood by anyone. Although many quake restoration organizations and volunteer workers from various cities in Japan and other nations came to his evacuation site and provided thoughtful psychological and physical support, he never felt understood by them. Later, when we began to work together, he told me, tearfully, that he was not able to trust people, especially people who came from a town less severely affected by the earthquake, or from other cities that had been exposed to similar disasters. He said, "I pretend to be nice to them, but I do not like them. Don't get me wrong. I think that they are wonderful people and I really wish I could accept their sympathy without conflicts, but I can't. Someone talked about how the quake attacked their towns; someone told a story of his grandfather and the a-bomb. But they don't have anything to do with my experience at all. I sensed that they were proud of their own experiences, and I felt deeply distressed by this attitude. I felt that they had sneaked into the special world that I am most proud of."

My patient was not able to voice these feelings for a long time, because he believed the people he met were well-intentioned and attempting to support him. He retreated into his painful pride, keeping a superficial relationship with others while the uniqueness of his traumatic experience both rankled and supported him, and sustained a sense of being in a cruel world. While the subjective experience of this patient is not generalizable to all survivors of the Great East Japan Earthquake, this example indicates the process through which the uniqueness of a traumatic experience is used by the traumatized person to maintain their individuality, at the cost of being alienated from others.

Of course, it is not only traumatic experiences that are unduplicated. Many events and phenomena in the human world emerge discretely and fortuitously. Starting at birth, and even prior to birth, all human experiences are personal and unique (Togashi, 2014a, 2017a). A particular man and woman meet in a certain way, their sperm and egg join at a particular moment and a baby is born in particular circumstances at a particular time. These particularities come from contingency in the world, and the reasons for them are inexplicable, but that, by itself, does not keep people from seeking to share their unique experience with others and making their shared experience the core of a sense of being human among other human beings.

Stolorow (2011b) posits an intersubjective basis of individual selfhood. He refers to Zahavi's (2005) delineation of three distinct concepts of self: the Kantian self, the narrative self, and experiential selfhood, which is considered to be primary to the "mineness" of experiential life. Stolorow suggests that Zahavi's tri-part concept neglects intersubjective contexts that promote the experience of mineness, and maintains that individuality in a human being is rooted "in shared recognition and understanding of our common human finitude" (Stolorow, 2011b, p.67). In Stolorow's perspective, a sense of individuality emerges in the intersubjective field in which each person's absolute uniqueness is a shared component of this common human finitude.

I believe that the absolute individuality of being born in this world leads to a sense of fundamental worth through the act of sharing and making sense of that individuality with others (Togashi, 2014a, 2014b, 2017a). Under healthy circumstances, parents enjoy talking to their babies about how they were born and have grown with the parents; even adoptive parents recount to their children the story of how they found each other and have been together, to their mutual pleasure. Having a sense of individuality and being with others are not mutually exclusive; rather, they are embedded in the intersubjective context.

Traumatized patients, on the other hand, wish to maintain a sense of being human *at the cost* of being with others. Such patients worry that they will be deprived of the uniqueness of their experience if they recognize another's experience or accept being recognized. Why, and in what context, does the uniqueness of one's experience become a traumatized individuality? And under what circumstances can it come to be shared with others and rightly used as the core of a sense of being human?

A key to answering these questions can be found in circumstances in which an *unspoken reality* leads to the recognition of differences among people. In the case of Hideki, the patient who participated in the group process for survivors of parental abuse, he felt it difficult to speak about the painful and often embarrassing experiences related by each member or to hear comments from them about his own painful stories. He felt that their abusive experiences were very different from each other, and inaccessible to him. Some members were physically abused, while others were sexually abused. Some members were almost killed, and others had never been physically struck. Hideki worried that to say something about their pain would only humiliate them further; he was afraid of being criticized by them for his shallow understanding, as he himself felt critical of their comments. The essential part of the pain of each member's experience was always a taboo for them.

My patient who survived the Great East Japan Earthquake was aware of more complex differences; he saw that volunteer workers and survivors were in different positions. Survivors' displaced condition made for ongoing issues, while the workers' experiences were temporary. Even within the survivor group, positions varied: some had not lost anything or anybody, some lost everything; some lost everything but had obtained considerable financial support from the government or a related company; some were severely wounded in the earthquake, and some had not suffered any injuries but no longer lived in their own houses due to radiation leakage; some, fortuitously, had not been in the region on the day of the earthquake and some had been in the middle of the disaster. In the group, however, they did not feel that they were allowed to speak about the most delicate part of their experiences which led to their division, even if they shared their stories. The survivor I treated felt envy toward survivors from other regions, because he believed that they had received large damage payments from Japanese national and local governments, and from the company that ran the nuclear facility. My patient never voiced this envious feeling publicly. He felt it as a taboo, although he thought everyone knew of the disparities, and he saw that other traumatized people, like himself, could not stop wondering if the person sitting next to them had received better or worse compensation.

As discussed in Chapter 5, traumatic events often divide communities, people, and the world into "my side" and "the other side," so that a traumatized human mind is also inevitably divided. This division is created by an unspoken reality, around which people organize the sharing of the essential part of their suffering. This unspoken reality strengthens a painful pride in each survivor, based on a sense that expressing the uniqueness of each one's traumatic experience would only increase the division further. In such a circumstance, there remains an invisible and intrusive element in the intersubjective field even when people share their stories.

Intersubjective taboo

It is well known that traumatization is associated with silence. In a beautiful and historic presentation in Kyoto, Japan, Orange (2018) describes how traumatization remains in silence and dissociation, which is often passed down through generations and expands into society and culture. She described the suffering of Ludwig Wittgenstein, who was not allowed to speak about his siblings' suicides, and how he was torn between the need to make personal confessions and the claim that "we must be silent." She states:

> The family required that the dead ones be no longer mentioned. Their spirits of those who departed had to be silenced, in a process my intersubjectivist teacher Bernard Brandchaft called "pathological accommodation" (Brandchaft, Doctors, & Sorter, 2010)—this means we sacrifice our own truth and self-experience to maintain needed bonds—and Leonard Shengold [called] "soul murder" (Shengold, 1989). Escape from this system of traumatizing malignant

> narcissism (Shaw, 2014; Turco, 2014) was impossible. Ludwig, the philosopher, fled to England, returning primarily to disinherit himself (Monk, 1990), by giving away his vast fortune after his father died. But he said little about his suffering, keeping silent.
>
> *(Orange, 2018, p.3)*

In this presentation, Orange (2018) illustrates many dimensions of silence surrounding traumatization. Some traumatizations are repressed in a Freudian way. Some are culturally and historically dissociated, and remain not only in an individual mind but also in a cultural and societal context. Some are simply kept silent.

Unspoken reality, I propose, does not refer to a repressed fact that may be discovered through a Freudian analytic procedure, but rather to a perception that both participants are aware of and have already shared at a certain level but have not spoken aloud. Neither does it refer to dissociation or "unformulated experience" (Stern, 2010), both of which mean that one part of a subjective experience is disavowed or disconnected from another. In unspoken reality, both participants are aware of and can access the experience. Their reticence is an *intersubjective taboo* (Togashi, 2016a), an unvoiced connection between two participants.

An intersubjective taboo, which works against being in touch with the essential aspect of traumatization, remains unspoken to protect the vulnerability of participants and the group. The shared perception remains unspoken as long as the relationship remains too vulnerable for it to be verbalized. In this sense, this taboo renders each member withdrawn into traumatized individuality, losing a voice with which to share the core elements of their suffering, and creates division among people between "your pain" and "my pain." At the same time, this taboo creates a bond and prevents a participant from absolute isolation from social connection—but as Orange (2018) describes, it is organized at the cost of their own truthfulness.

Authentic honesty and human suffering

How can this traumatized individuality be transformed into a sense of being human with others? How can we make the unspoken spoken?

Contemporary self psychological and intersubjective systems theorists agree, despite using different terminologies, in emphasizing the importance of honesty in psychoanalytic treatment with traumatized patients (Stolorow, 2007, 2008, 2011a; Brothers, 2008; Jaenicke, 2008; Carr, 2014; Togashi & Kottler, 2019).

They argue that fundamental human connectedness is organized around the intrinsic commonality in our existential makeup, and is rooted in authentic responses to human vulnerability, impermanence, and finitude in human existence. When people are forced to face human vulnerability in themselves, they often shut their mouths and avoid voicing their emotional experience. The intersubjectively shared taboo emerges as a manifestation of the particular traumatized vulnerability which seems to shake the very foundations of our humanity. These theorists suggest that the quest for open and honest dialogue about the taboo creates a space that does not threaten the uniqueness of their patients' experiences and allows patients to share those experiences with the analyst. "Ultimately, it is essential that the therapist (and patient) carefully observe and articulate how the 'unspoken' has transformed into authentic honesty in the therapeutic dialogue. Without this [they] believe a patient's recovery and transformation is superficial" (Togashi and Kottler, 2019, pp.328–329).

Carr (2014) discusses his work with a soldier who returned from the battlefield with severe post-traumatic stress disorder, after having participated in dehumanizing actions. As Carr strove to be empathic with the soldier, who recounted, in lurid detail, how he had killed insurgents and others in combat in Iraq, Carr experienced himself being unable to continue to listen. Carr recognized that he was threatened by his patient's descriptions, and that he had lost his authentic voice regarding his own sense of vulnerability. At that point, he said to his patient, "I don't talk about your pain because I feel helpless against it too. Your pain is overwhelming to me" (p.122).

Carr suggests that a therapist who works with a patient like his should not deny or disavow their "being-toward-death" but should maintain an honest acknowledgement of human finitude. Such an "authentic solicitude" helps the patient who has suffered exposure to an inhuman environment feel himself once again as being human. Carr's spontaneous, authentic response succeeded in making their psychoanalytic work a dialogic and relational home for traumatization. Carr states:

> Kinship-in-finitude also obligates us to recognize and bear together our differences. The qualities of our limits are unique to us. They make up our individual qualities, how we know each other. In the sense of divulging the shared and unique qualities of our finitude, authentic solicitude obligates us to care for the other as a unique human being, and can form the basis of friendship, love or a psychoanalytic attitude or ethic.
>
> *(Carr, 2014, pp.123–124)*

In this description, Carr suggests that the reason authentic solicitude obligates people to care for each other is the awareness that the suffering of the other in their presence is their suffering, too. When a human relationship becomes less human, people refuse to accept their suffering as their own and make it the possession of the other.

Tolstoy's *The Death of Ivan Ilyich* (1886) teaches us the difference between a deceptive kindness and an authentic solicitude. In a July 1981 interview, Kohut discussed this novella and described how a dying human being might long to have an honest relationship with another. Kohut emphasizes that, without such a connection, the person's life would be dehumanized. At the time of the interview, Kohut was in the middle of his ten-year fight with lymphoma, which ultimately ended in his death. Kohut lied about and hid the fact of his illness, and feared any authentic connection with others regarding the matter. Some researchers have mentioned that Kohut may have seen himself in Tolstoy's story (Strozier, 2001; Togashi & Kottler, 2015).

Tolstoy's hero, Ivan Ilyich, has lived a bourgeois existence and now finds himself dying from an incurable, unexplained illness. Although the people around him recognize that he is dying, they take pains never to acknowledge the fact, assuring him that he looks fine. Surrounded by dishonesty and deception, Ilyich cannot experience himself as being human. His only relief is afforded by a servant who stays with him and gives him the gift of a sincere voice. This story indicates that a traumatized individuality can only share an honest voice when the other displays an authentic attitude toward reality and human vulnerability. In the story, it is not because the servant mirrors his suffering that Ilyich experiences himself as being human, but because the servant sees Ilyich's suffering as his own.

The transformation process described in Tolstoy's late masterpiece could be seen as a process of making an individual uniqueness into a shared finitude. As in the two clinical examples cited in this section, we hypothesize that this process proceeds through an analyst's openness or "authentic honesty" about an unspoken reality. This process is examined in the following case vignette of Miyuki, a female patient with keloid scars on her face from burns in her childhood, who was first introduced in Chapter 3.

Case vignette—Miyuki

Miyuki was a computer engineer in her late twenties with whom I worked for eight and a half years, face to face, on a once-a-week basis. She initially came to see me complaining about a conflict relationship between her parents. She said that her parents were always quarrelling, her mother resentful of her husband's preoccupation with business and her father angry at his wife's manipulative behavior.

Two things interested me at the beginning of our work: first, although Miyuki's main complaint was about the relationship between her parents, she herself did not seem bothered by it very much. Rather, she felt herself to be outside the conflict; even when her parents and her brother argued with each other, she was rarely a target of their anger.

The other item of significance was Miyuki's facial scar. When she was four years old her kindergarten caught fire and she suffered severe burns, resulting in wide keloid scars on the left half of her face. Miyuki had undergone multiple plastic surgeries and had learned how to apply makeup skillfully enough that the scar was not immediately apparent to a passing glance, yet it was clearly visible to anyone who looked her in the face. They saw a refined young lady with a disfiguring scar. Significantly, Miyuki did not mention the scar at the beginning of our work.

It was not until several sessions after we started that Miyuki came out with the story of her scar and how her parents treated her differently because of it. She did not like her parents arguing with each other, but what was more disturbing was that they treated her with kid gloves and did not argue *with her*. She said that her parents had never admitted that they gave her special treatment because of her scars. She felt frustrated by this. In her adolescent years she would angrily ask them to treat her as a normal girl, but they continued to claim that they did not care about her scars at all, and that she should not be so sensitive about them because how she looked was not what mattered. Miyuki also knew that her mother often cried, tormented by a sense of guilt about her daughter's scars. All the family members were sensitive about Miyuki's appearance but never spoke openly about the subject; it was an intersubjectively shared taboo.

For our first two years, the main theme in Miyuki's therapy was her difficulty in talking about her emotional experience in session. She spoke cheerfully and airily in my presence and did not like to show weakness or vulnerability. Although she talked about many traumatic experiences that had happened to her, such as her burns and being bullied at school for her scar, she never cried. She sat up straight in her chair and kept her gaze straight ahead, rarely turning her face away from me. When something in the session made her feel vulnerable, she either kept silent or changed the topic. She had many social relationships with both men and women, but was afraid of being emotionally intimate. She revealed that, in her childhood and sometimes even now, she reminded herself not to hide her face and not to cry, no matter how nasty the remarks were that people made. She emphasized, "I will not be defeated by my fate. I have to live with the scars, but I don't think that it is a big deal."

At one point, I said to her, "It is understandable that you feel it difficult to talk about painful experiences, but tell me, what it is about me specifically that might have made you feel reluctant to reveal your experience?"

She answered, "It has nothing to do with you. I know you listen carefully to me and you understand what I say very well. It is me. I am afraid of touching my pain."

"Are you saying it is not related to me at all?"

"Don't get me wrong. I think that I am lucky to have you as my therapist. You are smart, kind, and very professional. But I don't think it matters much who you are, as long as you are professional."

Such dialogues often left me feeling alienated and isolated, even when Miyuki and I were actively talking. She determined what she needed to talk about, how she needed to talk and when she would stop talking. I felt that there was no space for me to engage. I felt myself to be a replaceable object, which led me to ask Miyuki who I was to her.

Miyuki told me, "I know I need you. I need someone I can talk to about my experience … I can't talk to the stones in the road."

"So, it should be a human, but it does not have to be specifically Koichi Togashi."

"I hope this doesn't hurt you, but … to be honest, no. You do not have to be you. I think that there is no one who could share my pain, which is very personal. To be more precise, I do not want to share my pain … it is mine."

My response was, "This is ironic. Your pain is unique and very individual, but the person you want to talk with does not have to be a unique individual. Anyone would be fine for you, as long as it is not an animal."

Miyuki recognized that she had confined herself in her own world by avoiding sharing any personal feeling with others, although she often complained about others' lack of understanding about her pain. She said that her withdrawal protected her from malicious remarks and from the painful and intrusive gaze of others. She knew, however, that this withdrawal also made her feel alienated and isolated. She was caught in a vicious circle.

One day, she came into my office visibly upset. She was breathing quickly, although she pretended to be fine. I asked her to explain what had happened. At first, she was hesitant to talk but finally opened up.

Miyuki said that she had stopped by a bank on the way to my office. While sitting in the waiting room, she happened to pick up a pen that had rolled past her feet. When she turned to face the young man who seemed to be the owner, he glanced at her face and, startled, dropped the pen again. Miyuki realized that her scarred face had alarmed him. Later, she passed the man as he was talking with a "beautiful young lady," and overheard their conversation. Not realizing that Miyuki was there, he said, "I was so scared by her face … I thought she was some kind of ghost or something."

Miyuki told me that she was deeply distressed, and she hurried into the bathroom at the train station to check her appearance. She was relieved because no tears showed on her face, but she was shocked by the fact that her heart was beating so rapidly. She did not think of herself as a person who could be distressed by such events.

"But, I was okay. I didn't cry … see?" Miyuki looked at me and smiled. Neither of us spoke for a moment. Then, she stopped smiling at me and shouted, "Don't look at me like that! I said I am fine!" At that point, I realized that I had made a grimace of pain, and that I myself had almost cried from feeling *her* pain. She cried for the rest of her session, almost twenty minutes.

Next session, she came to my office and said, "I have to say something about last week."

"Yes, I felt sure that you would."

"I saw my pain on your face. It said everything about how I felt. I could not avoid my feelings because I witnessed them on your face …"

Her using the word "face" surprised me because, until this moment, she had skillfully avoided saying it throughout her analysis. It was the first time that she had attempted to get over her weakness and be in touch with a part of her pain. It demonstrated her bravery.

Following that incident, Miyuki was able to talk about her feelings more deeply and emotionally, and allowed me to share her suffering. She was no longer alienated and isolated from me, even as she became more vulnerable.

In the fourth year of her therapy, Miyuki became more curious about how I felt about her and came to pay more attention to my own facial expression.

She said, "I like that I can see my feelings on your face. I had thought that I knew my own feelings, but your face tells me that I don't. I've discovered that your face tells me everything."

"How do you feel about my face?" I asked.

Miyuki smiled and said, "Well, it is easy for me to read. You are a person who cannot hide how you feel. Your face shows everything inside of you. I feel that I don't need to even 'read' your face … you are … No, your *face* is very honest." Miyuki and I laughed together.

Through this process, I came to recognize that my face expressed my attitudes honestly, no matter what I said aloud. When Miyuki tearfully revealed that as a child, she had been given instructions by her mother on how to kill herself if she chose, she looked at me and said, "I see tears in your eyes." All I could say was, "Of course there are."

One day, she told me about a dream in which her viscera collapsed and large amounts of blood thrown from her mouth. She associated this dream with childbirth, but she was scared and disgusted by it. I thought there were two meanings in the dream: one potential meaning referred to something negative, which could be a manifestation of her traumatic experience or temporal psychotic retreat. Another possible meaning, however, was more positive, i.e., that she was having a new experience. I only mentioned the second meaning, feeling that I should keep our dialogues as positive as possible, and because she looked scared.

Next session, she came into my office with an expression that indicated that she was upset. She told me, "Last week, you tried to be nice when we talked about my dream, didn't you?"

I said, "I admit that you are right. Probably I wanted to keep you happy, since you seemed scared by the dream."

Miyuki opened her eyes wide and smiled, "I like your honesty."

I said, "I like your honesty, too. When I came into my office, I immediately recognized that you were upset. Your face told me everything. Now we can both speak honestly with one another."

Honesty was of paramount importance to Miyuki. She talked about growing up aware that other people were not being honest with her. People said polite things about her appearance in an attempt to spare her pain, but they only made her feel isolated, segregated, and alienated. With tears welling up in her eyes, she said, "There is always something unspoken in my relationships, even with close friends. They are nice and kind to me, but I cannot see their real faces. I know that they are concerned about my scars, but nobody mentions them. The closer I get to them, the more I feel disconnected."

I told her, "They did not talk to you in perfect honesty, which probably felt like they were not treating you as a real human."

Honesty came to be the key word between Miyuki and me, as she allowed herself to become more open and vulnerable.

During this time, I recognized that I harbored feelings of guilt about *not* having scars on *my* face. Why did I have to feel guilty? Why was it a problem for me to simply say, "I am just lucky?" When I asked myself this question, I realized that it was only by chance that Miyuki had ended up with scars on her face; otherwise, her face might have been mine. I could have been Miyuki and Miyuki could have been me, and she had to take responsibility for her own life, being born in a world of contingency.

Following my realization, Miyuki began to talk about her inability to be involved in a romantic relationship with a man, an inability which had lasted all her adult life and which she had never been able to address with anyone.

One day, she began our session expressing dissatisfaction with her life. As she spoke, she looked down at the floor, and then, after about fifteen minutes, suddenly stopped talking. She remained silent a few minutes, then looked up into my face and asked, "I am ugly, aren't I?"

I was stunned into silence for a moment. As described in Chapter 3, a tangle of responses came and went in my head: "No, you are not ugly," "You don't have to worry about that," "What made you ask me about this question now?," "We should not deny this issue, but I think you are beautiful." I thought of all these answers and more in a few seconds, but in the end I said nothing. In fact, I thought that Miyuki was attractive enough, but it is also true that her scar was prominent. Her intense gaze made it clear that I could not gloss over the moment.

The few seconds of silence seemed like many long minutes. I could not speak, but simply and slightly nodded once. She did not reply.

Miyuki usually began a session by mentioning some feelings and thoughts she'd had in the previous session. In many cases, she referred directly or indirectly to a sense of anxiety and tension she had experienced in my presence. A week after Miyuki had asked me if she was ugly, she began the session with a remark about her feelings in the previous session but expressed it in an unusual way: "I don't want to talk about my feelings in the last session. You know the reason. Don't ask me anything about my feelings last week … I can't say anything. But what I can say now is that I no longer feel nervous here. I don't know why, though."

Miyuki requested that we not interpret what might have made her feel less nervous in session, but she appeared to be comfortable talking openly about painful experiences and events in her life. Her openness about her own life helped me to engage with her vulnerability and weakness. I felt it easier to envision her life, which I had thought was very different from mine.

Six months after the session in which we had discussed her appearance, I had a chance to ask her how she had felt about my attitude at that time. She said that she was ready to talk: "I was shocked by your confirmation of my word. But it was good because you were honest. People always try to be nice, but it is a lie … That was a moment of honesty and it made me feel better about my life … I once said that you did not necessarily have to be you. But now I feel that you are irreplaceable, a very special person."

"I am happy to hear that I am no longer 'Mr. Therapist,' I am Koichi Togashi, a human being who is meaningful to your life."

Since this period, Miyuki gradually opened herself to greater intimacy with others and finally found a relationship. Toward the end of her therapy, Miyuki and I shared an understanding that one of the big issues we had struggled with was bravery. She told me that she lacked the courage to face her scars, which were a manifestation of pain and suffering. I lacked the courage to acknowledge that the pain of her suffering was beyond my understanding. I recognized that I felt guilty about not having scars on my own face, and feeling guilty, I separated us into different categories: traumatized and non-traumatized. By doing so, I denied the shared cruelty and impermanence of the world. Once I admitted these qualities, I had to face the fact that it could have been me who had the scars on my face, and that it was totally random and coincidental that it was she who was exposed to that traumatic event. Three sessions before the end of her therapy, I shared my understandings. Miyuki listened to my statements and finally said, "I think I will keep fighting forever, but I don't think I need my armor anymore. Thank you."

Discussion and conclusion

Miyuki was traumatized not only by her facial scars and related insults, but also by seemingly compassionate treatment when people were overly solicitous of her emotions. Like Hideki and the survivor of the Great East Japan Earthquake, she did not enjoy sharing her emotional experience with others. She alienated herself by not seeing others as unique human beings, while she withdrew into the painful pride of her unique experience, her traumatized individuality. Even after years in treatment, she was still able to maintain that it did not matter who her therapist was. She protected her individuality by avoiding being together in a fully "I-Thou" relationship. In the therapeutic relationship between me and her, there had remained an unspoken reality, a taboo: how both of us experienced her face.

How was Miyuki's traumatized individuality transformed to a sense of being human with me? It was in the moment when she asked me if she was ugly and I nodded that she stepped forward to a sense of being human with others. At the same time, my reflection on my own sense of guilt became a recognition of the impermanence and contingency of the world. We shared, at that moment of nodding, the absolute uniqueness of this impermanent world. In this process, her sense of the uniqueness of her suffering was transformed into a sense of the shared uniqueness of the world.

And did this process proceed because of my authentic honesty? My answer is no. I do not deny that our therapeutic work touched at the periphery of honesty or authenticity. It was when Miyuki was gradually coming to be in touch with her own vulnerability that she happened to have the incident at the bank. Later, in my office, I was almost in tears from feeling her pain. Seeing my expression, she shouted, "Don't look at me like that." She might have seen hope and dread (Mitchell, 1993) in my face, and no doubt, she was familiar with "poor you" looks. But she also said that she welcomed my honesty and might have been hoping for a potential new relationship with me.

Since that event, Miyuki and I have talked about honesty in my face and in human relationships. But had I been honest? Had she really experienced us being honest? As discussed in Chapter 3, this case vignette indicates that this was not necessarily so. From the beginning of Miyuki's therapy, there was a big question between us about "how she looked." We knew that we both thought it wrong to avoid the issue, but we were afraid of touching on the topic. In session, Miyuki sat up in front of me and looked straight ahead. The scars were clearly visible. I knew she was concerned about how I felt about her appearance, and she knew that I was concerned about how she experienced my gaze, but we did not speak openly and honestly about our concerns.

The time came when, finally, she asked if she was ugly and I nodded. Was this a moment when my honesty came through? Unlike Carr's example, I did not mention my own vulnerability or my fears of talking about how her traumatization appeared in her face. I only nodded, with the recognition that I could have been her in another universe. This was not authentic solicitude. There is no question that I shared the unique quality of our pain, but what made it possible was only my throwing myself into the unique tragedy of the contingent world, in which, as discussed in Chapter 5, there are no distinctions between a person with scars and a person with no scars. This was not honesty in the sense indicated in Carr's example.

Neither did I display "sincere honesty" at this moment in the usual sense, as discussed in Chapter 3. Although I nodded, I did not simply think that she was ugly; I did not express my thoughts and feelings completely, nor did they match my action. What changed Miyuki's withdrawal into traumatized individuality was, rather, that she and I surrendered ourselves to the world as it is.

In my understanding—from the decolonizing perspective that makes up this book—what made this transformation possible was our *makoto* kind of sincerity. *Makoto*, discussed at length in Chapter 3, is a Japanese ethical concept of sincerity, not merely a sincere state of mind but a reflection of a cosmic tide of Nature which is at all times transforming and changing.

From an aesthetic standpoint, according to Reasoner (1990), *makoto* is "the fundamental truth contained in the essences of things and self, and their ultimate unity" (p.483). The key features of this aesthetic are purity, brightness, and uprightness of the minds and things which see themselves as they are. In this sense, he claims, "*Makoto* functions at a fundamental level and preserves a type of objectivity; what the poet [artist] apprehends of things in *makoto are essences*, not private or idiosyncratic visions" (p.483; italics in original).

If we apply this lens to my psychoanalytic work with Miyuki, we can say that it was the *makoto* kind of sincerity, more than authentic honesty or sincere honesty, that unfolded in an intersubjective field, a field that is continually transforming and changing. Miyuki and I surrendered ourselves to the tide of this intersubjective field. We abandoned personal values and thoughts at that moment and forgot social and professional roles. She just asked and I just nodded.

8

A SENSE OF "BEING HUMAN" AND TWINSHIP EXPERIENCE

As my colleague and I have written previously (Togashi, 2012, 2014a; Togashi & Kottler, 2012a, 2012b, 2013), a traumatized patient often describes "not feeling human," or feeling that they have lost a sense of being human in a relational context. For example, a sexually abused female patient described herself as "a toilet bowl," an object into which someone else's sexual impulses were disposed. Although this patient said she did not feel like a human being, she recognized herself as belonging to the human species, and therefore as "a human." However, in this relational context, she did not experience herself as being human or being treated as human.

This type of anguish is not described by traditional psychoanalytic terms such as *functional deficit, disruption of ego structure, fragmentation of the self,* or *splitting of self- and object representation*. It goes beyond a malfunction of the internal psychic structure to the collapse of humanness. It is the erosion of confidence in being a human in this world. What is it about a traumatic event that might make a person lose a sense of being human, and how might we help the person regain the sense of being human through psychoanalytic work?

Since Freud (1896, 1905a, 1906) downplays the psychological effect of trauma in the etiology of neurotic symptoms, traditional psychoanalysis, with few exceptions, has failed to address trauma and traumatization. It is only very recently that psychoanalysis has accepted that trauma has a profound impact on the human mind, and tried to illustrate its subjective meaning. Self psychologists and intersubjective systems theorists have developed "trauma-centered theories" (Brandchaft, 2010; Stolorow, 2007; Brothers, 2008; Togashi, 2014a, 2015; Togashi & Kottler, 2012b, 2013, 2015, 2018) that directly focus on the existential anguish coming from the lack of a sense of being human. These authors' discussions go beyond the illustration of pathological effects (such as dissociation, multiplicity of self, or symptoms of PTSD), to attempt to articulate a psychoanalytic process in which the traumatized patient is again able to organize a feeling of being human, and they show how a sense of *twinship—a sense of being a human among other human beings* – can evolve within a dyad (Togashi & Kottler, 2012b, 2013; Togashi, 2014a).

In this chapter, I attempt to illustrate the ways in which a person experiences him or herself as being human, or being treated as human. I also work to develop a model for understanding and treating a patient who feels a lack of this sense. The chapter includes a review of the psychological literature on humanness and humanity, and psycho-biographical research on Heinz Kohut. It was in his last ten years, while he was battling the lymphoma that ultimately killed him, that Kohut began writing about humanness and the meaning of being human (Kohut, 1981, 1984, 1985). Atwood and Stolorow (1979) maintain that a psychoanalytic theory and the theorist's life are engaged in a dialectic relationship, and it is in that spirit that I attempt to explore the effects of the agony of cancer on Kohut's theory of humanness.

In order to shed light on Kohut's thinking, we first examine the experiences of cancer patients in the terminal phase of their disease and the attendant challenges to their sense of being human. Second, we review the ways in which psychoanalysis describes a sense of being human, and how Kohut (1984) employed the term "twinship" to describe a sense of "a human being among other human beings." Through this examination, we can delineate the essential elements of an experience of oneself as being human, and how those elements are organized. Finally, we'll see a model of the experience of being human from a contemporary self psychological perspective.

Although the exploration of a sense of being human includes philosophical and ethical issues, this chapter focuses on practical issues in psychoanalytical work with traumatized patients and attempts to examine how such patients, along with their analysts, can articulate the psychological meaning of the lack of a sense of being human.

The humanistic trend in clinical ethics of terminal care

We begin with the ways that "humanity" or "being human" is addressed in the clinical ethics of terminal care. Many philosophers and medical professionals have studied the fundamental aspects of human dignity in terminal care (Pfeifer et. al., 1994; Nuland, 1994; Pastrana et. al, 2008; Hermansson & Ternestedt, 2000; Lannamann et. al., 2008). The requirements for human dignity indicated by these studies vary depending on the context under discussion, such as patients' self-expressed needs, necessary knowledge for mediational professionals, clinical ethics, etc. For example, factors in improving quality of life of terminal patients, Hermansson & Ternestedt (2000) focus on issues of symptom control, self-determination, social relations, self-image, synthesis, and surrender. Ragan, Wittenberg, & Hall (2003) suggest that palliative care must engage "existential issues of meaning, relationships, autonomy, guilt, dignity, and communication," and Lannamann et. al. (2008) maintain that the essential element of communication between medical professionals and patients who face the end of life cannot be generalized, but they see honest conversation, self-determination, existential issue of meaning, necessary information including expectancy of life, and spiritual care as fundamental aspects of human dignity.

In my review of these articles, the fundamental aspects of human dignity that most theorists in this area share can be summarized as follows: 1) self-determinism, 2) honest and sincere emotional connection with others, and 3) the meaning of one's life given by others after death. This section looks at the ways in which a dying person attempts to preserve human dignity through these three aspects, although I would like to emphasize that the elements of human dignity vary and cannot be limited to these three.

The Advisory Board to the Congress of the Federal Republic of Germany on "Contemporary Medical Ethics and Law" compiled an interim report (Deutscher Bundestag, 2004), in which the *advance directive* (*Patientenverfügung*) appears as a significant tool in considering how a patient can die *humanly*, i.e., with human dignity intact. An advance directive is an oral or written declaration of intent with regard to medical treatments. It is given *in advance* by a patient who maintains decision-making capacity, to affect decisions to be made *in the future,* when he or she will have lost that capacity. Unlike a will or testament, it is not intended to control activities after the patient's death, but to control the time before death.

In reference to advance directives, the Advisory Board (Deutscher Bundestag, 2004) identifies the right of self-decision as one of the most important human rights. This view is rooted in Western ethical values of autonomy and self-determination. Still, it is clear that dying patients often do not feel themselves at the center of initiative or decision, but instead experience themselves as desperately helpless. This anguish is outside of any specific cultural background.

Discussion about advance directives is significant in clinical ethics because, as human beings, we are inherently disturbed by the thought that the direction of our lives and being may be decided in ways beyond the scope of our knowledge. This fear is particularly stressful today, when people are required to manage an increasingly complex array of medical technologies and legal issues.

Honest and sincere emotional connection with others is also an important theme for traumatized patients, since they often experience themselves as isolated or disconnected from others. Nuland (1994), a physician engaged in end-of-life care, explored ways in which a human could die humanly. Not only was he a clinician who treated dying patients, but he also witnessed the deaths of family members—an older brother and an aunt—from cancer. Through these experiences, he was led to think about the meaning of human dying. According to Nuland, caregivers and loved ones err by not facing the end-of-life phase of an illness directly, when they avoid talking about death or about the patient's physical condition. Inevitably, patients recognize their future, and friends know about their fates. By not talking about the shared truth, friends and relations make patients feel more alone when being with them. Nuland (1994) describes this phenomenon as follows.

> We convinced ourselves she didn't know, though we sensed that she did, as she must have convinced herself we didn't know, though she must have known we did. So it was like the old scenario that so often throws a shadow over the last days of people with cancer: we knew—she knew—we knew she knew—she knew we knew—and none of us would talk about it when we were all together … In this sense, my Aunt Rose died alone.
>
> *(Nuland, 1994, pp. 244–245)*

Another illustration, for Nuland, comes from Leo Tolstoy's (1886) short novel, *The Death of Ivan Ilyich*. In this story, a well-to-do judge named Ivan Ilyich suffers a devastating illness, a gradual physical implosion, during the course of which he is treated in his house. As he endures the process of dying, he feels alone, despite the many doctors, friends, and relatives who come to see him and attempt to care for him. For Ilyich, the essence of his experience with others is a lack of honesty. His friends and relatives know that Ivan's condition is very serious; but no one tells him the truth and say only that he looks fine. They fail to share his sense of fear and despair. The only person who allows him his humanity is a simple servant, one who is not intelligent but is honest with him.

This novella illustrates two causes for the loss of a sense of being human: first, loneliness and the lack of emotional connection with the people around Ilyich; second, a sense of despair at the collapse of his own body. As we will see, it is hardly coincidental that Kohut (1981), too, referred to this novella in discussing the meaning of being human.

Nuland (1994) also addresses the third requirement for humanity in dying: the meaning of life given by others after death. He maintains that the subjective experience of death differs depending on the way in which other people give meaning to one's life. If patients can find meaning in the lives of people who will live on after them, they can experience themselves as being human even though they die. However, as Nuland (1994) points out, many dying patients fail to find meaning in the future after their death and cling to hopes for extended life, often relying on medically invalid therapeutic methods which, ironically, often prevent them from achieving calm in the face of death.

The humanistic trend in psychoanalysis

Due to his materialist and objectivist bias, the concepts of "being human" and "humanity" were not sufficiently addressed in Freud's clinical and meta-psychological theories of psychoanalysis. Many subsequent theorists, however, have addressed these themes, often in ways that are antithetical to the Freudian mechanical and biological view of human beings (see for example, Frankl, 1946; Boss, 1963; Binswanger, 1963; Fromm, 1959, 1979, 1989, 1994). The humanistic trend remains in vogue and some theorists (Friedman, 1982; Lichtenberg, 1985; Meissner, 1985; Sass, 1989; Frie, 2011; Stolorow, 2012; Orange, 2015) point out that research on the meaning of humanity and the sense of being human has received renewed interest in recent years.

At issue is not whether Freud denied or rejected the consideration of "humanity" in psychoanalysis. Rather, as Boss (1963) points out, Freud struggled to find a way to view his patient as a whole human being. While he banished some colleagues and followers who criticized his theory and sought more holistic, religious, or philosophical understandings of human beings, in other cases he enjoyed dialogues with analysts with religious and philosophical leanings, such as Binswanger and Pfister (Frie & Reis, 2001; Frie, 2011, 2012). Living in an age that celebrated natural science and objectivism, however, his effort to find a way of depicting the whole human being drifted into an atomistic perspective in his clinical technique and meta-psychological theory.

As described in Freud's theory, being human is, in a certain sense, simple and mechanistic; the human animal is inherently controlled by sexual impulses or aggressive drives, and the development of a human being is a history of training and controlling these maladaptive impulses. To be a *human* human being, one must learn to repress and disavow these impulses, as well as organize the ego which functions independently from them. The ego is fully structuralized through the successful resolution of the Oedipus complex (Freud, 1913, 1923b, 1927, 1930).

With such a model in place, Freud's theory was skeptical about humanism and psychologically grounded ethics. In this theory, the essence of humanity is "intelligence" or "knowledge," and a person is human to the extent that he can control his primitive, beast-like nature. Freud's model suggests that a human being should not be afraid to see the bestial aspect of his unconscious—understand it, engage with it, and control it.

Yet Freud's attempt to address the whole of human nature did not prove to be a total failure; his theory suggests the analysand is a human being who struggles to find him or herself in loving interaction with others. Freud's followers expanded the humanistic elements of his theory, hidden by the scientific rationalism in vogue at the time, to a theory of whole human being. For example, Erick Fromm (1989, 1994), known, along with Horney and Sullivan, as one of the Neo-Freudians, writes that the "experience of humanism" is that:

> ... as Terence expressed it—"Nothing human is alien to me"; that I carry within myself all of humanity; that, in spite of the fact that there are no two individuals who are the same, the paradox exists that we all share in the same substance, in the same quality; that nothing which exists in any human being does not exist in myself.
>
> *(Fromm, 1994, p.77)*

Sullivan (1953), Horney (1950), Fromm (1959, 1979, 1989, 1994), Boss (1963), Binswanger (1963), and many others describe human development as being embedded within a social and environmental context. They all emphasize that a human existence emerges in the intersubjective or interpersonal field, in circumstances which include intimate care, love, and authentic dialogue.

These theorists overlap with Kohut's view of being human, which is organized in the field of selfobject experience. He states:

> Throughout his life a person will experience himself as a cohesive harmonious firm unit in time and space, connected with his past and pointing meaningfully into a creative-productive future, [but] only as long as, at each stage in his life, he experiences certain representatives of his human surroundings as joyfully responding to him, as available to him as sources of idealized strength and calmness, as being silently present but in essence like him, and, at any rate, able to grasp his inner life more or less accurately so that their responses are attuned to his needs and allow him to grasp their inner life when his is in need of assistance.
>
> *(Kohut, 1984, p.52)*

For Kohut, self-experience always emerges within the context of the other's responsiveness. In other words, selfhood involves both authentic being and experiences of relatedness. The idea is most clearly described in his definition of the twinship experience, "being a human being among other human beings" (Kohut, 1984). In my view, the twinship experience is organized by two people who are "mutually finding himself and not-himself in each other" (Togashi, 2012). This is an experience organized between emotionally connected people who recognize similarities and differences vis-à-vis one another (Togashi, 2012).

A significant difference between Fromm and Kohut lies in Fromm's emphasis on self-awareness. For Fromm (1989, 1994), human experience is organized after a person is aware of being in this world; the experience of being human is "that of man's self-liberation by optimal self-awareness; of the attaining of well-being, independence; of the capacity to love; and of critical, disillusioned thinking, of being rather than having" (Fromm, 1989, p.64). For Kohut, the emphasis is on being connected to other people—whether consciously or unconsciously—and emotional connection, or empathic relationship (Kohut, 1959, 1981), is more significant for one's sense of humanity than awareness.

Sass (1989), in his excellent review of the humanistic trend in psychology and its philosophical background, classifies four essential qualities of human psychology: freedom, uniqueness, privacy, and self-transparency. Sass named *freedom* as a human quality and states:

> Influential humanists (or proto-humanists) like Allport (1961), Rogers (1961), and Bugental (1965, 1967) argued that the human being's most distinctive and important feature was the capacity for volitional choice. Lip service may have been paid to such constraining factors as culture, nurture, or biological inheritance, but far greater emphasis was placed on the capacity for free will, which was generally seen as capable of outweighing these deterministic factors.
>
> *(Sass, 1989, pp.438–439)*

Uniqueness emphasizes the idiographic nature of personality, prizing the uniqueness of each person's experience. This view also leads to an emphasis on self-actualization and the need for individuation, for being oneself as a person. *Privacy*, related to uniqueness and freedom, fulfills a significant function in Sass's human psychology, emphasizing subjectivity and the inwardness of human reality.

The fourth aspect of Sass's humanist psychology, *self-transparency*, refers to self-consciousness. "It implies a vision of human nature as involving a form of fundamental and unquestionable self-knowledge" (Sass, 1989, pp.444–445). It is a stance that suggests that all of a person's personal data are available to her awareness, and can be openly owned by her.

Sass (1989) includes Harry Guntrip (1971), George Klein (1976), Heinz Kohut (1977), Donald Spence (1982), Merton Gill (1983), and Roy Schafer (1983) as part of the humanistic trend in psychoanalysis. He argues that their works can be categorized along the lines of his four qualities of humanistic thought, and illustrates how these four facets are addressed in their writings.

While Sass and other theorists have addressed essential facets of the human experience, they have not directly addressed the problem of the patient who feels himself as *not human*. Psychoanalysis is a clinical theory for a psychological treatment; it aims to make a patient experience more ease. What I want to draw attention to, going forward, is not the definition of humanity, but the patient's struggle to experience him or herself as being human and the need to be treated as human. It is important for psychoanalytic practice to see this struggle and this need; this is the essential focus of our efforts when we face traumatic experience. According to Togashi & Kottler (2012a), a part of Heinz Kohut's legacy for psychoanalysts is a way to address this challenge.

Kohut's "being human" and twinship experience

Kohut's self psychology began with his attempt to establish a therapeutic relationship with patients with narcissistic personality disorder, and to explore a therapeutic intervention for them (Kohut, 1968, 1971). First, he classified the narcissistic relationship into two types of selfobject (originally, self-object) transferences: mirror transference and idealizing transference (Kohut, 1971, 1977). He describes these as the ways through which patients attempt to experience themselves as vital, cohesive, and secure. According to Kohut, selfobject transferences are not pathological themselves, but are indispensable for achieving a certain sense of the self; they constitute nutrition for a psychologically healthy life. The reason these transferences often look pathological or troublesome is due to the patient's extreme yearning for such experiences and consequent demand for immediate gratification. Yet Kohut sees the narcissistic relationship as the way to maintain the sense of self.

It was in his 1968 paper, "The Psychoanalytic Treatment of Narcissistic Personality Disorders—Outline of a Systematic Approach" that Kohut introduced the word *twinship* to refer to an archaic form of mirror transference. He originally thought that mirror transference occured in three different forms, depending on the developmental stage of the grandiose self, and saw twinship as a subtype. By 1984, he came to see twinship as an independent selfobject relationship or experience, as a third way to maintain the sense of self, alongside mirroring and idealizing.

In the process of this therapeutic and theoretical exploration, Kohut (1977) came to recognize that what he had found was not a way to treat "narcissism," but an understanding of how the "self" or "self-experience" can be organized or transformed. This understanding evolved into his "psychology of the self" or "self psychology," in which the main topic is the way of experiencing the self.

Still later, however, as my colleague and I have pointed out (Togashi & Kottler, 2015), Kohut, through a series of studies of twinship experience and transference, shifted his perspective from "the psychology of the self" to "the psychology of being human" (Togashi, 2012; Togashi & Kottler, 2012a, 2012b, 2013), defining twinship transference as the "need to experience the presence of essential alikeness" (1984, p.194). Similarly, he expanded twinship to define it as "confirmation of the feeling that one is a human being among other human beings" (Kohut, 1984, p.200). Now the twinship experience became an essential aspect of humanity, of being human. Because of his early death, Kohut's thinking on this topic could not evolve further, but I believe that at the time of his death, "experience of the self" was no longer his main theme. By then, "being human" or the "meaning of being human" had become the essential topic in his psychoanalysis.

Kohut's life

Heinz Kohut was born in Vienna on May 3, 1913, the only son of a wealthy and musically inclined, assimilated Jewish couple. According to Strozier (2001), Kohut was thoroughly exposed to the rich and varied traditions of German art, thought, science, history, and music throughout his childhood. He studied medicine at the University of Vienna from 1932 until 1938. In the wake of the Nazi invasion in 1939, Kohut immigrated to England, arriving first at a refugee camp and later staying at an uncle's home for a time. It was on March 4, 1940 that he finally entered the United States. He chose to reside in Chicago and, after graduating from the Chicago Institute, began his career as a psychiatrist, devoting himself to the psychoanalytic field as a clinical analyst.

The 50s and 60s were golden years for ego psychology in America, and Kohut was a well-known and respected ego psychologist, as Anna Freud appreciated (Strozier, 2001). His lectures in ego psychology were widely praised for their logic and clarity (Strozier, 2001), and he served as president of the American Psychoanalytic Association from 1964 to 1965.

From the 1970s onward, Kohut began to develop his original ideas that often sharply departed from the ego psychological tradition, and eventually bore fruit in his theory of self psychology.

I date the beginning of Kohut's theoretical shift at sometime around 1971, when he was diagnosed with lymphoma. This was shortly after publishing his first book, *The Analysis of the Self.* In this book, Kohut attempts to adhere to the tenets of Freudian psychoanalysis as much as possible (Stolorow & Lachmann, 1980; Lee & Martin, 1991; Strozier, 2001) and, despite the expression of many original ideas, never challenges Freud explicitly. After 1971, however, Kohut begins to bring his own ideas to the fore and often confronts the ego psychological perspective directly. As a result, he was exposed to widespread criticism, and was expelled from the legislative council of the Chicago Institute and other committees.

In the ten years after his diagnosis, Kohut witnessed his own body collapsing, losing function, deformed by edema and illness. He lost energy but continued to devote himself to writing, and lectured as often as possible. On October 4, 1981, he delivered a final lecture at the University of California, Berkeley, then returned to Chicago where, four days later, he died.

In the course of Kohut's life, he was condemned as non-human twice (Togashi & Kottler, 2012a, 2015). First, after the German invasion of his country, he was no longer identified as a citizen, but as a Jew, which, under the Nazi administration, meant "less than human." According to Strozier, Kohut did not think of himself as a Jew, but as a person in the great German cultural tradition. Nevertheless, when the Nazis invaded, they saw Heinz Kohut as neither German nor human. A Nazi occupied his house, he was disenfranchised, and his right to sit for his medical examinations was cut off.

The second loss of humanity for Kohut occurred with the onset of his cancer and the collapse of his body. Strozier (2001) revealed that Kohut tended to hide his illness from the people surrounding him, and that he often lied about his condition. I believe that it was due to a preoccupation with protecting his own work that Kohut lost honest and authentic relationships with others. The theoretical shift of twinship transference and experience took place during this ten-year period.

Being human in Kohut's writings

In a series of interviews undertaken by Strozier (himself both an historian and a psychoanalyst), in the last eight months of Kohut's life, Kohut implicitly maintains that the goal and moral purpose of psychoanalysis is to explore the meaning of humanity. When Strozier asked Kohut to describe what history means to psychoanalysts, Kohut stated, "it [history] serves, like every other human activity, to support life as we cherish it, to make us more human and to maintain our feelings as human beings so that we can be responded to by others and understood by others" (Kohut, 1981, January 29, p.221).

In the same interview, Kohut (1981) criticized traditional psychoanalytic ethics coming from Freudian drive theory, which sees a human being as inherently beastlike, reclusive, and not open to transformation. He stressed that contemporary psychoanalysts have to articulate the fundamental anguish of being in the human world and understand its ultimate sense of loneliness.

> The worst—and I think I said this most concisely in the final reflections of *Advances* (1980)—is to find oneself in a predominantly non-human environment. This is the dreadful fear of our time, to be shot off into space and to be all alone. There is a wonderful symbol of psychosis in dreams. It is that you get out of the gravitational attraction of earth and are by yourself forever. Even a hostile empathic environment is vastly preferable to an indifferent one.
>
> *(Kohut, 1981, January 29, p. 222)*

This description goes beyond the functional problem of self structure, which Kohut (1971, 1977) originally attempted to explore. The "dreadful fear" Kohut describes has to do with the sense of loneliness and the question of whether or not the "I" exists as a human being. It is a fear organized around a sense of being human, not the lack of the cohesion of the self. By this point, as my colleague and I (Togashi & Kottler, 2015) suggest, Kohut's psychology had already gone beyond the psychology of the self and into the psychology of existential anguish about being in the human world.

For Kohut, a sense of being human or being part of humanity has to do with temporal continuity in one's being:

> Man tries to support human life, including psychological life. This is behind everything I have to say. The historian supports the continuity with the past so that people can feel better about themselves.
>
> *(Kohut, 1981, February 12, p.226)*

However, *feeling* oneself as being human is different from simply *knowing* that one *is* a human. Referring to the period before and during the war, Kohut says:

> Millions of people at that time understood and were able to live in accordance with Nazism. It came at enormous cost to their humanness and their ability to understand other people's sufferings and feelings. They switched from feeling human themselves to feeling like the only humans or almost the only humans.
>
> *(Kohut, 1981, March 12, p.252)*

From this description, it is clear that even if one knows oneself to belong to the human species, one would be unable to have the sense of being human without others with whom one has a shared history. Only when people can put themselves in the shoes of others and feel that others can walk in theirs can they co-create the world and history. For Kohut, the sense of being human comes from finding oneself in empathic connection with other human beings and experiencing a temporal continuity through those emotional connections.

This notion is consistent with our discussion (Togashi & Kottler, 2013) of Kohut's shift of emphasis in the definition of twinship from a sense of essential alikeness (Kohut, 1971, 1984) to a sense of being a human among human beings

(Kohut, 1984). We asked ourselves why Kohut kept using "twinship" even after this shift, and concluded that

> an essential quality of a sense of being "a human among humans" in a twinship tie relates to the way in which the two people experience their meeting and their being together as coincidental, but also, significantly, as irreplaceable.
>
> *(Togashi & Kottler, 2015, p.159)*

I believe that a healthy mother enjoys talking to her child about how she experienced her pregnancy and delivery, and how she has been together with the child. Through this attitude, the mother expresses her joy about encountering her baby as coincident, but in a significant and irreplaceable way. We conclude that a sense of being human, for Kohut, is "finding meaning in the ways in which they are born, and their ways of being among other human beings" (Togashi & Kottler, 2015, p.166).

Connectedness with the authentic other

Kohut describes another way in which a person feels himself as being in a human environment. In his interview of July 1981, he cites the same tale that Nuland found so illustrative, Tolstoy's (1886) *The Death of Ivan Ilyich,* and talks about what makes Ilyich's death human or inhuman:

> … when somebody tells a dying person what an example he is to him when he will have to cross that barrier, that line, and how he admires him for the way in which he handles and faces this trying moment, the last moment of his life, a dying person hearing that may die proudly. The opposite occurs when the selfobjects retreat from the dying person and abandon him, either by not visiting him anymore or by emotionally walling themselves off. This is so beautifully described in *The Death of Ivan Ilyich* by Tolstoy. In that story everybody goes about his way blissfully, not wanting to be reminded of death. The wife does this and the friends do that. The man would have died miserably had there not been one selfobject, a servant or serf, who stayed with him and massaged him and at least stayed in some degree of emotionally meaningful contact with him. This is what made the dying bearable.
>
> *(Kohut, 1981, July 16, p.264)*

For Kohut, a sense of being with human beings can be organized through connection with an authentic and honest other. This type of emotional interaction does not necessarily mean a positively colored relationship or compassion for each other, but it does mean that perfunctory care or a lie disturbs a human relationship, while being in the presence of the other who exists simply and authentically can create meaning. Through the relationship with the authentic other, a person can make their being in the present meaningful and can link their past to the present.

As Strozier (2001) reveals, Kohut struggled to conceal his lymphoma and physical condition from the public, and he was not able to be connected to the other in an authentic way. David M. Terman was a psychiatrist who was a candidate at the Chicago Institute in the late 60s and had been in supervision with Kohut for almost four years. He (Terman, 2013) testifies that Kohut never talked about his own illness or about his childhood. According to him, Kohut was very concerned about how he looked in his lectures and always held strict rehearsals beforehand. What he showed others was not himself, but an idealized self.

Nevertheless, Kohut's reference to *The Death of Ivan Ilyich* in describing the feeling of being human represents his yearning for an authentic relationship with others, which he knew that he was unable to have. According to Anna Ornstein and Terman (2013), long before he was diagnosed with lymphoma, Kohut displayed a reluctance to talk about himself, although when the floodgates opened, he could monopolize the conversation in a way that often turned people off. From this we conclude that his difficulty in having honest, emotionally meaningful relationships with others was not due to his lymphoma. Rather, his lymphoma made him recognize his yearning.

Finding hope in passing on something to the next generation

In what way was Heinz Kohut himself able to maintain a sense of being human while he faced his death? It is striking that he went to Berkeley only four days before his death to speak at the self psychology conference. Kohut's enthusiasm is confirmed by Ornstein and Terman's testimony that he was preoccupied with expanding awareness of his self psychology in the mental health field, and with passing on his ideas to the next generation.

At the end of his life, Kohut (1984) described twinship as "the little girl doing chores in the kitchen next to her mother or grandmother; the little boy working in the basement next to his father or grandfather" (Kohut, 1984, p.204). Here, twinship manifests itself in an individual's effort to look for a successor (Togashi, 2009; Togashi & Kottler, 2015). For Kohut, an individual's effort to educate others is often based on the yearning for a person whom one can experience as essentially alike, a person in whom one can find oneself. Kohut (1977) describes this feeling as that of a boy's father who "looks upon him proudly as *a chip off the old block*" (Kohut, 1977, p.234; italics added). Kohut sees the twinship experience as yearning to pass on a part of oneself to the other living in the future, which is exactly the nature of Kohut's strong yearning towards the end of his life. This yearning represents a proof of the legitimacy of his being, and a hope for his life in the future.

For Kohut, it is the hope of passing on something significant to the other in the next generation that creates the environment in which people have empathic relationships with others, feel themselves as continuous in being in this world, and feel their lives as meaningful. The other does not necessarily live now; it might be a person living in the future. I believe that Kohut himself, in his selfobject fantasy, might have been able to have meaningful relationships with people who have not yet been born. They are the successors through whom Kohut could keep his theory alive (Togashi, 2009). Through this experience, Kohut could expand his own life into the future and articulate the meaning of his life.

Process of experiencing being human

In this chapter, I have tried to illustrate how a sense of "being human," as manifested in Kohut's twinship selfobject experience, can be defined as a psychological state in which a person feels an emotional tie with others and makes sense of temporal continuity in her being. I argue that such an experience can be organized through sharing with the other about how the person was born and how she has been with the other, through an authentic and honest relationship with others, or through the hope of passing on something significant to the next generation.

Kohut's life was not always tranquil. Strozier (2001) attests that Kohut's mother, Elsa, had an unstable personality; she was moody, full of ups-and-downs, and manipulative in highly intrusive ways. Kohut grew up identifying with German culture and art, but was expelled from his country by the Nazis and defined as non-human. It is not difficult for us to imagine that Kohut would have been highly ambivalent about "how he was born and how he has been with others." As Strozier (2001) and Terman suggest (personal communication, 2013), in his last years Kohut longed for honest emotional connections with other people, but had difficulty achieving them. They said that Kohut rarely talk about his childhood, and often lied about his physical condition. Rather, what he felt was probably an absence of such an environment.

Kohut had tenacity and endurance, and propounded his ideas even though strongly criticized by traditional psychoanalysts (Strozier, 2001). He was preoccupied with creating himself in the other, a twinship experience that he describes as "passing on talents and skills to the next generation" (Kohut, 1984), and the effort made him feel alive. Indeed, in the speech delivered four days before his death, Kohut seemed to acknowledge that his ideas would have an influence on the future of psychoanalysis and believed that they could be broadly applied in other mental health fields (Kohut, 1975, 1982).

In Figure 8.1 the process of experiencing oneself as being human is shown as the connection of a person's subjective experience from the past to the present, from the present to the future, and the realization of a person's experience in the present. Through this conjoined process, people can feel empathic relationships with others, continuity in their own being, and make sense of the meaning of their own lives. This is not a static process but an active, mutually influenced one. When one part is foreground, the others are background, and the sense of being human is not dependent on all three parts being fully organized at any one time.

How can this model be applied to our clinical work with the patient who complains about the lack of a sense of being human? We can build our psychoanalytic work on these same themes: how the therapist and patient happened to

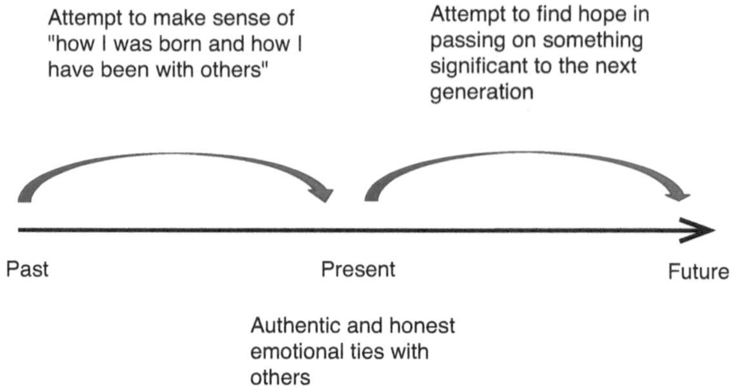

FIGURE 8.1 The process of experiencing being human in Kohut's self

meet and have been together, how both parts of the analytic dyad experience their relationship as honest and authentic, and whether or not the therapist and patient can find themselves in each other. The model implies that when patients fail to have these experiences in a therapeutic relationship, they may experience the process as re-traumatization, by losing the experience of being human.

This is consistent with the study in which we illustrate that traumatized patients may be anguished by the simultaneous need for sharing experience with the next generation, and the need for ending the traumatic experience in their own generation (Togashi & Kottler, 2013). In such a situation, patients are deadlocked by their opposed efforts to recreate their traumatization in the next generation on the one hand, and isolate traumatization from the next generation on the other. Trapped in this dilemma, honest and authentic emotional ties with people in the next generation, or the hope of passing on something significant to the next generation, are lost.

We have discussed the relationship between ways of experiencing contingency or coincidence and the relational trauma (Togashi, 2014a, Togashi & Kottler, 2013). Contingency, which has a long history as a topic of philosophical discussion (Kuki, 1932, 1935; Rorty, 1989), has a profound effect on a sense of being human. Traumatization is usually caused by an event that occurs in one's life without rational reasons, and traumatized people feel it is difficult to make sense of the experience. They ask themselves, "why?" but they are severely challenged to find a reason. In my understanding, the tragic nature of human experience comes from the contingency of the world. One of the aims of analysis is to articulate organized experience in the contingent world and find a way to feel it as a moderately reasonable place. To live in this world is to find possibility for humanity within the irrational, in a space between necessity and contingency.

What is a sense of being human?

In the preceding pages, we have examined the ways in which people experience themselves as being human, including being treated as human by others. We concluded that a sense of being human can be organized through sharing with others about the contingency of the world; one's perception of where we came from and how we have been with others; through authentic and honest relationships with others; or through a hope of passing on something significant to the next generation.

We have also suggested, in this discussion, that these human processes represent a person's effort to survive the irrationality of the world, which is *a priori* included in trauma. For survival in the traumatized world, a person is required to maintain a delicate balance between a sense of certainty and uncertainty. While one has to recognize that there are no definitive explanations for why one is born in the traumatic world, one can still share this human fate with others. The potential for finding meaningful experience in an irrational world, and perceiving a hopeful future, is a significant gift of being human.

Finally, we can examine these conclusions through the decolonizing lens of the psychoanalytic zero, which suggests that people's efforts to find this sense of being human, the means of surviving trauma, paradoxically *creates* a wounded and traumatized world. People seeking a sense of being human divide the world between humanness and inhumanness. They define the world in which they feel connected with others as "human," and the irrationality of the world as "inhuman." But irrationality is an inherent quality of the universe; it is only human beings who identify that which is human or inhuman.

As discussed in Chapter 5, some Eastern ethical perspectives view the human world as a traumatized world that emerges when people fail to surrender themselves up to the cosmic tide of Nature. Trauma divides the world into categories, which must be identified and named. Naming the world creates all human experience, including anguish, suffering, happiness, and well-being. For these Eastern ethics, human suffering, in particular, is created by one's preoccupation with difference—with naming, categorizing, and choosing between observed phenomena, instead of surrendering to the universal tide which precedes and underlies all human distinctions.

Kohut was preoccupied with humanness. He theorized and defined the twinship experience as a sense of being a human being among other human beings. Through his twinship idea, he explored how human beings are born and connect with others. He was preoccupied with having authentic and honest relationships with others, while he avoided talking about his own illness or his childhood. He was preoccupied with passing on his own ideas to the next generation. But he could not let himself be himself, and we could say that his preoccupations—his efforts to experience himself as being human—created his traumatization. We can also say that those same efforts were only brought into his life in the wake of his traumatization.

The paradox that emerges from applying *the psychoanalytic zero* to *the psychology of being human* suggests that, while the struggle to maintain a sense of being human is a natural human response, needed to survive the irrationality of the world, this human attitude itself makes the world traumatized. Further, it is these traumatized divisions that create culture, politics, arts, and all other facets of human society.

We also need to recognize that we have a prejudice embedded within a Western perspective, in which our seeking humanness and human spirituality is seen as sublime and valuable. We cannot escape from our preoccupation with seeking a sense of being human.

I should point out that this chapter itself is written out of my own preoccupation with a sense of being human and my own acculturation with Western values. Even the humanistic trend in psychoanalysis itself includes inhumanness. Creating and discussing a psychoanalytic theory, and our attempts to find a way to help a traumatized patient are all ways to avoid surrendering ourselves to the cosmic tide of Nature.

In my understanding, there are two ways to survive the irrationality of the world: surrendering ourselves to emptiness (as discussed in the previous chapters), and finding a sense of being human. But the two ways are not necessarily mutually exclusive; rather, our humanity may emerge in the moment when both ways are entwined. A sense of being human cannot be found without surrendering ourselves to emptiness; surrendering ourselves into emptiness is not possible without the effort to find a sense of being human.

9

THE PROBLEM OF UNCERTAINTY

The future of psychoanalysis

The subtitle of this chapter, "The Future of Psychoanalysis," is taken from a 1975 article of the same name by Heinz Kohut. The article was originally presented in 1973 at a sixtieth birthday dinner party in Kohut's honor at the "Psychoanalysis and History" conference in Chicago. In his talk, he discussed the value system expressed by psychoanalysis and his expectations for psychoanalysis in the future. He noted that psychoanalytic work has become embedded in today's social values and ideals, and claimed that psychoanalysts are often required to be aware of the degree to which their own personal values and ideals are affected by social values and ideals.

Kohut wrote *The Future of Psychoanalysis* shortly after he was diagnosed with lymphoma and following the publication of his first book, *The Analysis of the Self* (1971). The article was, in a sense, his declaration of independence, a significant step toward establishing his own psychoanalysis. He was becoming freer and more open about expressing his own theories, and, in the article, demonstrates that he is no longer concerned with how traditional psychoanalysts feel about his ideas.

Kohut began his article with two personal stories. The first was an account of his return to Vienna after his exile during the Second World War; the second, a memory of seeing Freud at a railroad station at the beginning of the war, as the older man was leaving Vienna to emigrate to England. Kohut used these experiences to describe the passing of an era and the loss of idealized figures, pointing out that social values, ideals, and interpersonal relationships were very different for people living in Freud's day, and that subsequent generations had been forced to re-evaluate and create new values and ideals. For Kohut, the 70s were a pivotal time. Most psychoanalysts educated by Freud had passed away and the new generation was no longer constrained by older ways of psychoanalytic thinking:

> What I am speaking about is the moment when Freud who, as an archaic image is still living on concretely in those who serve as substitutes for him, will

> die a second time, i.e., will finally die. I am speaking of the moment when the community of analysts will realize that they have not inherited an identification, goal-setting as well as curbing, but have been given the legacy of an opened door, allowing entry into the vast unexplored area into which the first explorers could make only a few halting steps.
>
> *(Kohut, 1975, p.328)*

In Freud's time, "the highest ideal of psychoanalysis" (Kohut, 1975, p.329) was to find the truth behind manifest phenomena; by the time of Kohut's Chicago talk, the ideal had become finding an idealizing object through which a person could maintain "the exhilarating expansion of the self" (Kohut, 1975, p.336). The first ideal is based on a world view in which there is an objective truth within a psychological phenomenon, and a rational understanding of the unconscious is achieved by an observing ego. The latter view presumes that people seek to maintain a sense of self by connecting to something stable or reliable, and that a person can find a sure and certain subjective experience within a human relationship. Kohut relates this shift in the value system to changes in society and its interpersonal milieu. In Freud's day, people lived surrounded by family members and faced emotional conflicts due to over-stimulation and over-involvement. By the time of Kohut's article, people faced an attenuation of human relations and, as a result, experienced a need to find someone through whom they could regulate their grandiose fantasies and idealizations in order to maintain a sense of self.

Kohut implies that psychoanalysis, too, would change its focus, from unmasking a truth in order to produce definitive answers, to exploring the way people find idealizable figures in a world of tenuous human relationships. He states:

> The full integration of [Freud's] ideals may allow the analyst of the coming generation to become the pacesetter for a change in the hierarchy of values of all the branches of science concerned with man, through a shift of emphasis from a truth-and-reality morality toward the idealization of empathy, from pride in clear vision and uncompromising rationality to pride in the scientifically controlled expansion of the self.
>
> *(Kohut, 1975, p.334)*

For the future of psychoanalysis, Kohut was neither overly pessimistic nor optimistic. He believed that psychoanalysis has many possibilities within itself, including structures for self-renewal. He stressed that psychoanalysis provides a perspective, represented by the Oedipus complex, for understanding how a new generation overcomes the emotional conflicts that come with confronting the values of the older generation. As the new generation brings new values, it creates a space for revolution and transforms the field.

What are the essential social and interpersonal values of our time, a time of profound social change, increased reliance on information technologies, terrorism, violent tribal and non-state conflicts, climate change, and other disruptive world traumas?

One answer is that there are no *essential*, generally agreed-upon values, and that the human species has survived in the world without them for all of history. But today, we have become more and more sensitive to the unpredictability, unknowability, and uncontrollability of our society and human relationships; we seem to be overwhelmed by a sense of uncertainty in the human world. No one can predict what will happen tomorrow, no one knows what is true, and no one is sure where society is headed. Some suggest that as modern technology develops, with more information coming in and more decision-making turned over to automated systems, the world comes to be felt as progressively more uncertain.

Although Kohut (1975) saw the interpersonal milieu as attenuated, he did not seem to view the world as being as uncertain and contingent as we feel it today. He writes, "once the old ideal has been replaced by the new one, the new one is now held to be as perfect and absolute as had been its predecessor" (p.324), implying that a new ideal takes over the old one and forms the basis of a value system. Where he saw a change of value systems, what I see today is the unpredictability, unknowability, and uncontrollability of society, and of any value system—in other words, a world felt as uncertain with no widely shared values and ideals.

At the time of this writing, *the sense of uncertainty* is a cutting-edge topic in the relational and ethical trends in psychoanalysis. Trauma-centered psychoanalysis based on the ethical trend explores the relationship between trauma and a sense of uncertainty (Stolorow, 2007; Brothers, 2008; Togashi, 2014a, 2014b, 2014c; Togashi & Kottler, 2019). These thinkers suggest that a sense of uncertainty is deeply connected to such existential trauma as genocide, nuclear bombs, and random killers. Though it would seem that there is nothing secure in human relationships, people still want to believe that the stranger sitting behind them will not stab them with a knife. In the face of tsunamis and earthquakes, we still want to feel that our lives are basically safe and secure. Healthy people are able to find a sense of certainty in relationships with others, even while they feel the larger world is uncertain (Orange, 1995; Janoff-Bulman, 1992; Kauffman, 2002; Togashi, 2014a, 2014c, 2014d).

Some relational and intersubjective analysts focus on the unpredictability and unknowability of the psychological phenomena psychoanalysts work on, and the unprovability of psychoanalytic theories and procedures themselves (Hoffman, 1998; Harris, 2011). Relational thinkers (Stolorow & Atwood, 1997; Miletic, 1998; Renik, 1998; Jaenicke, 2008), have discussed concept enactment, or implicit processes in human interactions. They say that we analysts are no longer able to hide ourselves behind anonymity, or so-called neutrality, nor can we passively accept what the patient says. Deconstructing traditional theories of meta-psychology and psychoanalytic techniques, they point out that the traditional perspective is not a universal truth that allows clinicians to explain all human developments and therapeutic processes. Rather, they maintain that all therapeutic relationships are uniquely organized at a certain moment of a certain dyad between a certain patient and a certain analyst, and that the therapeutic process is ever changing, moment by moment.

These theoretical discussions, in both the relational and ethical trends in psychoanalysis, ultimately ended up in the same place. Trauma-centered psychoanalysis, which focuses on how traumatized people divide communities, society, and people in order to have a sense of certainty, offers a treatment model in which a patient comes to live with a sense of *uncertainty*. The model emphasizes that a patient and an analyst share human finitude or contingency of the world in "a relational home" (Stolorow, 2011a). The world and others may be eternally incomprehensible, but human beings can emotionally connect with each other only through acknowledging human finitude and the contingency of the world. The relational and intersubjective theorists, who focus on the unpredictability and unknowability of our professional work and theories, require that analysts throw themselves into a sense of uncertainty, and live with it before they request their patients to live with it. As we say, "the patient can only go so far as the analyst is willing to go" (Frie, 2011, p.144). It is not until a therapist can live with a sense of uncertainty that a patient will be able to live with it.

So, what do we mean by "living with a sense of uncertainty?" Is it even possible, and if so, how can we do it? What does the problem of uncertainty mean for our psychoanalytic work with our patients?

My goal in this chapter is to address the problems of uncertainty and certainty that we face in our daily lives—personally, professionally, and in our psychoanalytic work. From a general discussion of certainty and uncertainty, we'll go on to examine the sense of uncertainty experienced through trauma. Finally, we'll discuss the problem of uncertainty in psychoanalytic practice.

Certainty and uncertainty

The world is not uncertain, although we experience it as uncertain. Neither is the world certain, although for the most part, we experience it as certain and predictable. The world always does what it does. If a tsunami kills 20,000 people, the world is no more or less uncertain, but we feel the world profoundly differently. If we focus on the tsunami's unpredictable influence on human lives, the world is felt as uncertain; but if we view the tsunami as evidence of the vulnerability of the human body, our perilous condition in this world is confirmed and felt as certain. It is only human beings—with ever-changing expectations, perspectives, and division—who name how and what the world is.

How do people experience the world as uncertain? If certainty and uncertainty are an artificial dichotomy, then it is either when people assume the world is *supposed* to be certain or when their belief about the world's uncertainty is sure that people experience it as uncertain. People who witness violent acts of terrorism, and therefore interpret the world as being an uncertain place, are somehow imagining a "certain" world in which people are not killed by terrorist attacks. Alternatively, there are those who loudly affirm, "the world is in chaos!" demonstrating the certainty of their perspective. Either way, uncertainty becomes another form of certainty.

Ironically, the more people seek a sense of certainty, the more they become sensitized to uncertainty; as people realize a kind of certainty, the world's felt uncertainty stands out. For example, if a city successfully establishes a system that reduces traffic accidents by an order of magnitude, its citizens are all the more overwhelmed by a sense of randomness and uncertainty when a now-rare traffic accident does occur. As the world becomes measurably more predictable and certain, it feels more uncertain. Human history is a long narrative about the struggle to deal with the unpredictability and unknowability of the world. In all measurable ways, this 10,000-year story has moved in the direction of greater certainty and predictability. Ironically, however, people living today complain of "the uncertainty of the world," in spite of the technology that allows us to make more successful predictions than ever.

So, how we can help our patients to live with a sense of uncertainty? And first, how can we help ourselves to live with a sense of uncertainty?

Therapists' attempts to familiarize our patients and ourselves with an environment felt as uncertain are doomed to fail because as soon as we attempt to accept a sense of uncertainty, we recognize that we are seeking a sense of certainty. Further, the more a patient becomes accustomed to uncertainty, the more he or she is tied to seeking a sense of certainty. Not seeking a sense of certainty means bearing the pain and anguish of uncertainty, which only grows greater over time, and avoiding the pain means denying the possibility of certainty, which is the stance of a skeptical and pessimistic hermit.

Picture a patient who complains about the irrationality of society or the random nature of natural disasters, and a therapist who suggests that the patient should simply agree to live with a sense of uncertainty. Such a suggestion would be rejected and frustrate the patient further, because it comes from the therapist who is apparently comfortable in the certainty of his own suggestion. Intersubjectively, we would say that this therapist is preoccupied with certainty and the patient is required to relinquish the sense of certainty; the result is that the relationship becomes stuck with "the doer and done-to" (Benjamin, 2018).

Instead, what we can do is let this artificial division go. The world itself is neither certain or uncertain. The things we feel sure of are only sure to the extent that we can predict and understand them, and we are always already betrayed by them because there is no *prior consent* between people and the world (Togashi, 2017a, see also Chapter 6).

Psychoanalytic theory is also both certain and uncertain, trustworthy as well as untrustworthy. When a therapist experiences an analytic theory as certain, that is the same as saying that she is confident in her knowledge and wisdom. Certainty does not indicate how valid the theory is, but rather, how the therapist experiences it. Likewise, believing that a psychoanalytic theory is uncertain tells us nothing more than that a given therapist is certain of the theory's inaccessibility and unworkability.

So, what *does* exist in the absence of certainty and uncertainty? This is the moment without context, from which our psychoanalytic work emerges. In other words, the moment of radical encounter between a therapist and a patient, in which there is no pathology, no diagnosis, no need, and no theory to assign to the patient as yet. As discussed in the Preface, this moment exists not only at the very first encounter, but also in every moment of psychoanalytic work. The therapist who surrenders herself to the moment without context frees herself from the division of certainty and uncertainty and stands outside of any theoretical framework. Once we enter into the psychoanalytic process, however, we cannot escape from our preoccupation with certainty and uncertainty, because we use a predictive framework in order to interact with the physical world. The issue is not to figure out whether it is more correct to have no framework or a predictive framework, but simply to be aware of the preoccupation. Once we can see this process, perceived theory and perceiving therapist are no longer divided. They are wound around each other; theory and therapist are one.

Certain and uncertain aspects of trauma

If we surrender ourselves to the moment without the context of certainty and uncertainty, how can we work with the patient suffering from trauma?

At the experiential level, a traumatic event shows us two worlds simultaneously; a world felt as having something certain (which does not always mean something positive), and a world felt as having nothing certain. Traumatic events such as genocide make us feel that we live in a chaotic world without the hope of certainty, and simultaneously make us feel certain that the human world is one in which people are killed by others who were able to recognize them as human beings just days or weeks earlier. A tsunami helps us to recognize the sure and finite nature of our bodies, and simultaneously makes us feel Mother Nature as unpredictable. In a case of abusive incest, a girl may certainly experience herself as "something" her father desires, and she also finds the love she believed in to be untrustworthy.

While an actual traumatic event makes us experience the world we live in as being irrational, uncertain, and coincident, it also defines us to ourselves by dividing, categorizing, and naming the world. It helps us to see how we live, who we are, and how we are seen by others. When trauma destroys the order of our beliefs, it creates a sense of uncertainty; when it shows a way to see ourselves, it creates a sense of certainty, usually that something is "bad." The two sides of trauma are opposing faces of the same coin. Both provide a *Weltanschauung* by drawing a clear picture in a world that looks uncertain.

Traumatization, as discussed in Chapter 5, is defined as a division of the world, community, people, or society in the wake of trauma. A traumatized person comes to be preoccupied with identifying every event as "good" or "bad," "my side" or "the other," certain or uncertain. Traumatized people are no longer able to surrender themselves to the flow of the undivided universe. They are busy defining who or what is a perpetrator and who or what is a victim, and what aspects of their mind (sometimes, of course, all of it) have been shattered by what. There is no such thing as *nothing* for them, no co-existence or merging of categories.

This is a challenge we all face. Surrendering ourselves to the moment without division, between certainty and uncertainty, puts us in a vulnerable position. As Ghent (1990) says (discussed in Chapter 1), people who surrender themselves to emptiness are thrown off-guard. Without our social and professional preoccupations, and minus the artificial roles and constructions we rely on in our daily lives, we find ourselves in a state of radical vulnerability.

Certain and uncertain aspects of analytic work

We like to believe that the psychoanalytic theories we embrace are reliable and certain but, as some contemporary theorists (Atwood and Stolorow, 1979; Orange, 1995; Stolorow, Atwood, & Orange, 1999; Frie, 2017b) suggest, the psychoanalytic theories have been established in the context of specific and limited social and cultural values. Given that context, how should we understand our work and our patients' suffering?

It is widely known that Freud expected to see psychoanalysis accepted as a scientific model, and its developmental and meta-psychological models as universal truths of the human mind. He believed that all boys are destined to reach the Oedipus complex by a certain age, and all girls are doomed to fail to work through that complex. He was certain of his theory and devoted himself to affirming it. After his death, his followers took over the job of illustrating the universality of Freud's theories. Even among the next generation, who challenged Freud's perspective and established new perspectives which did not necessarily follow Freud's views (Rank, 1924; Jung, 1921, 1951), the aim was still to establish a universal theory of mind.

But, as we've discussed, psychoanalytic theories are not always useful for understanding non-Western patients, or even some Westerners. Some theories help us to find a certain and consistent pathological organization in a patient's mind (Kohut, 1977; Kernberg, 1975), but there are many patients we cannot describe or understand from a traditional psychoanalytic perspective. Contemporary thinkers, in particular, emphasize the uncertain aspect of our psychoanalytic theories. Some theorists argue that the stability of psychological illness is merely a myth (Mitchell, 1988; Kohut, 1971, 1980; Stolorow, Brandchaft, & Atwood, 1987, Gill, 2000). We know that psychological illness is context-sensitive, and that psychoanalytic phenomena (e.g., transference, repetition compulsion, resistance) are not substances but co-creations in a particular context between a particular patient and a particular therapist (Bacal, 2006, 2010). We want to believe that our psychoanalytic technique works when a patient improves, but it may be only coincidence (Togashi, 2014a). We often find ourselves unable to tell when patients get better what cures them or what makes them well.

The psychoanalytic model itself is neither certain nor uncertain. It is simply a perspective from which to see the world, or part of it, i.e., our clinical works and our patients' minds. But it is the therapist or patient who experiences the theory as being correct or incorrect, useful or off-target, certain or uncertain. And when they experience a particular psychoanalytic model as useful and certain, they often believe that their subjective experience indicates a universal truth.

At issue is in what context a psychoanalytic theory is experienced as certain or uncertain. As the clinical situation changes moment by moment, so is our subjective experience transformed. At one point, the therapist simply listens to the patient without concerning himself with theory; at another time, he is focused on applying a theoretical model to what the patient is saying. The key to understanding the context is the therapist's acceptance of his own fallibility and vulnerability.

When we affirm in our minds the certainty and rightness of a theory, we confirm our own rightness in believing in it. When a therapist says, "this theory is true," it is the same as saying, "my understanding is true." It's when we are not able to live with our own fallibility and vulnerability that we emphasize the rightness of the theory. When a patient wants to physically touch us, when a patient complains about the insufficiency of our understanding, or when a patient does not get better, we often retreat into theory and rely on the certainty of the rules the theory teaches us to follow.

Not knowing the certainty or uncertainty of our analytic theory puts us in a vulnerable position, but this vulnerability does not mean weakness. It is a radical vulnerability; another expression of the emptiness from which everything is born and to which everything is reduced. The psychoanalytic zero requires us to be in this vulnerable position when we see our patients, who are themselves afraid to be vulnerable. It is the only moment in which a patient and therapist are together in this universe without preoccupation regarding certainty and uncertainty.

Clinical example

A Japanese patient, Shoko, an intelligent and socially successful woman in her thirties, came to see me complaining about problems with her marriage of ten years, which she ended during the course of her six-year psychoanalytic psychotherapy. Shoko was frustrated by the fact that she could not find a definitive reason why she felt her marital life was so bad, though she was strongly convinced that it was horrible and traumatic. For Shoko, it was this absence of a bad event, i.e., *nothing*, that was disturbing. She knew that her married life was not what she believed it should be, but she did not know what the essential issue in her anguish was. She was convinced that something was wrong, but she could not tell what or how.

Shoko met her husband through a matchmaking arranged by his aunt. In accordance with her husband's wish, Shoko gave up her professional career when she married and devoted herself to housekeeping. Eventually, she and her husband had two daughters, who were nine and six years old at the time Shoko began therapy.

Shoko said she felt an extraordinary sense of hollowness and meaninglessness in regards to her marital life. She described her husband as unable to have an emotional relationship, and revealed that she could not remember a time when she and her husband laughed with each other.

Shoko's husband was a medical professional and earned a good salary, which he kept to himself, giving her a monthly allowance of a thousand dollars to keep their house. The amount was sufficient, but Shoko felt that her husband doled out this allowance in a business-like manner with no feeling of love. The husband had a little alcohol at dinner every night, drinking by himself and not talking with family members. Shoko did not feel comfortable with him when he was drinking. His behavior and demeanor were not violent, but his way of communicating with family members was emotionless, and Shoko said that their daughters never attached to him.

Shoko began her therapy speaking in a gentle manner, but without creating a space where I could talk with and for her. She gradually began complaining about her marital life with more intense emotional expressions of anger, humiliation, and sadness. The manner in which she spoke made it easy for me to understand how deeply she was wounded by her relationship, but I had difficulty grasping what actual events in her married life disturbed her. When I asked her to describe an episode when she felt distressed, she was not able to come up with any clear examples. She seemed to have difficulty characterizing her married life and was unable to verbalize the central cause of her distress.

Another troubling feature in her analysis was her obstinacy. She did not have the financial resources to maintain her sessions, but when I offered to reduce her fee, she turned down my suggestion in a definitive manner and insisted that she wanted to pay full price, as a matter of self-respect.

I had a hard time understanding both her obstinacy and the ambiguity of her distress. I did not feel the content of the problems with her husband was consistent with the intensity of her emotional expression. She said that she had not been treated by him as a human being, but I did not know what made her feel that way. I said to her, "Your sadness and humility and anger look very deep, and I believe that they indicate the intensity of the distress you experience in your life with your husband. But I feel some gaps between the severity of your expression and the episodes you describe." In response to these comments, she tried to relate in detail how her husband treated her badly, yet, as she talked about her husband's behavior, I felt certain that her husband had not done anything bad *to* her. I finally came to recognize that the issue was that he did not do anything *with* her, and that *nothing* meaningful was more traumatic to her than *something* horrible.

In the middle of her therapy, Shoko asked me to explain her husband's behavior. She said, "I believe that you can analyze my husband and solve his mystery." She reiterated that she was not able to determine how and why her husband's behavior was difficult for her, but she was certain he had been horrible. She maintained that nobody understood her distress because, to outside observers, her husband looked and acted perfectly gentle and normal.

I attempted to understand her motivation in asking me to explain her husband to her, but when I focused on her motivation, considering it as a defensive pattern she had created, she would not back down and continued to ask for my explanation of her husband's behavior. I found myself feeling annoyed, and thinking that it was this stubbornness that must have created the emotional conflict with her husband. I thought, at the time, that her stubbornness was the issue *we* needed to work through, but the longer I continued to see her request as *her problem*, the more depressed she became.

I finally recognized my error when she asked me, "Why do you always interpret my problem when I am asking you to interpret my husband's problem?" I recognized that not only was she unable to live with her vulnerability in a marriage that contained nothing meaningful, I was equally unable to accept *my vulnerability*. I dared not take the risk of analyzing her husband's behavior *in absentia*, assuming that the person with the problem was her, not her husband. When I denied her request by saying, "it is impossible for me to describe a person I have not seen before," I was facing—and avoiding—the same dilemma as Shoko, i.e, my vulnerability. My way of avoiding vulnerability was by interpreting her through the psychoanalytic theory which felt certain to me. But I came to understand that this was the issue we had to work on: that we both avoided our vulnerable state. I finally allowed myself to say something about her husband, even though I was unsure of my interpretation because I could not meet him in person. But the more I put myself into that vulnerable position, the more freely Shoko was able to talk about her own experience.

Five years after the beginning of her therapy, Shoko said that she understood the essential issue in her experience of her marriage and was able to verbalize what had made her distressed. She said that her husband did not seem to be interested in how Shoko and their children lived, nor did he share any feelings about her giving up her career, about her pregnancy, giving birth, or caring for their children. Her husband, who had met dozens of women in matchmaking meetings before her, did not remember how Shoko and he had met the first time. He spent a lot of time playing video games on his own. Shoko complained about the games, but the issue was not the games; it was that he neither paid attention to her nor invited her to join in playing. While Shoko described their sex as "sadistic," it was rather the case that it was affectless: she did not feel any sense of love or passion when they started or finished. Her husband touched her body without saying anything, made love, and went back to playing video games in the next room immediately after they were done.

Over time, Shoko and I came to share the hollowness of her marital life. Although Shoko described the relationship with her husband as "being treated badly," in fact, it was even less than that, and thus it was understandable that she felt that she was not treated humanly. She said that her husband treated her as a toilet bowl, not because he treated her in a sadistic manner, but because he did not see her as a human being. In one session, she said, "I tried to tell you how my husband was bad to me, but he was not even bad. I recognized that, to him, I am not a meaningful human being."

It was a significant theme for Shoko to understand why she expressed her experience in such a strong fashion; for example, describing affectless sex as "sadistic." She once related an episode involving a photo her husband had. The photo, which seemed to have been taken for medical use, was of a grotesquely deformed part of a woman's breast. Shoko told me, "I think that he brought it into our home because he wanted to show it to me. After I saw it, he wanted to make love with me. Do you see how humiliating that was for me?" My detailed inquiry, however, revealed that they had sex more than a month after she saw the photo, and we found that she had connected the two unrelated events to reframe their dispassionate, empty sex as a frightening and humiliating experience.

In our discussion, we came to conclude that her extreme expressions were her attempt to find a sense of certainty in her hollow life. Sadistic sex was more certain than unaffectionate sex, for a sadistic husband would expect an aversive emotional reaction and enjoy her expressions of pain. In other words, identifying her marriage life as sado-masochistic created a sense of certainty about her life. It outlined who she was and what her life was. Trauma made her aware of being in a "certain" world, and awakened this awareness with powerful emotional impact.

In the course of her therapy, Shoko decided to get a divorce. When she told her husband he reacted with malice, saying, "I don't think that you can live by yourself. You can do it if you want." In the process of negotiating the divorce settlement, he made unreasonable demands and often begrudged giving her money. Interestingly, his aggressive and manipulative attitude made her feel relieved. She said, "I can now clearly see that our relationship is problematic. Thanks to his harassment, I had the chance to confirm that my husband is the problem." Then she said that she had been like a new-born baby who did not know who she was, what the world was like, and what people were like. I told her that she could tell what the world she lived in was like as long as she saw visible negative features of her husband.

After her divorce, the next task for Shoko was how to address the "bad" in people. For Shoko, all men now became perpetrators and all women victims. Although she found a professional position, she was unable to continue in it. She attacked male colleagues for tiny mistakes and became intolerant of small failures by men, including me. As her aggressive attitude became more severe, I initially understood it as part of a process of mourning, working through the loss of her life and her marriage. My effort to understand her pain, however, did not succeed. She criticized me for the insufficiency of my understanding and my inability to say anything to sooth her painful feelings.

One day, at the end of a month, I forgot to give her a bill. She was furious and attacked me, saying, "you do not think I'm an important patient. That's why you forgot to give it to me." She said that all men were selfish and cold. I simply said that my failure made her feel sad and lonely, like her ex-husband had done. But she refused to understand, saying "you should know that you are not a good therapist. You may want to consult someone more skillful."

This therapeutic impasse continued for six months, during which time I came to feel more uncomfortable being with Shoko. In one session, she began complaining about a male colleague, who was not Japanese. In the process of her criticism of him, she became emotional and referred to him using a racial slur, which made me uncomfortable. In the moment, I said that this kind of statement was intolerable for me. "I understand that you are frustrated, but racial discrimination is not acceptable." I then told her about my own similar experience while I was in the United States, and how painful it was for me. She reacted with more aggression, but in the next session, she apologized for her actions. She cried and said that she had not been treated as a human being by her husband, but it was wrong for her to treat other people inhumanly. We shared the understanding that she had experienced discrimination at her husband's hands. She and I agreed that it is inevitable that we are treated by others inhumanly, and we treat others inhumanly, because we are all vulnerable human beings.

Toward the end of her therapy, Shoko and I discussed our encounter. She said that through this relationship she was able to understand the meaning of her experience with her husband. Otherwise, she might have remained suspended in an uncertain anguish. In this way, we discussed how we had been together in session.

One day Shoko talked about her not accepting my suggestion of reducing her fee, and said that she needed to be obstinate because otherwise she would have been overwhelmed by a sense of vulnerability. She asked me, "…how did you feel about me at that time? Maybe you felt me a drag, didn't you?" I answered, "No … I did not feel that way, I felt your being strong, as you described yourself. I believed that you would beat your husband in the end." She laughed and said, "I like your honesty."

Discussion and conclusion

Until she left her husband, Shoko had been frustrated by the fact that she was not able to identify the negative aspects of their relationship, even though she knew that her married life had not been successful. What our therapeutic work revealed was that their relationship had been so shallow that her husband did not even remember how he met her. There was nothing meaningful in her life with him.

Shoko did not experience physical or verbal abuse from her husband, but her married life *was* traumatic in the sense that her relationship to her husband was totally hollow. This is a good example of Kohut's idea of trauma arising out of nothing. As I discussed in Chapter 8, one of Kohut's most significant contributions is his perspective that an essential factor of human anguish is the sense of nothing (Kohut, 1981). He stressed that contemporary psychoanalysts have to articulate the existential anguish of living in the human world and understand its ultimate sense of loneliness.

At the end of his life, Kohut took a sharp turn away from the traditional psychoanalytic perspective. Traditional psychoanalysis hypothesizes that psychological illness derives from "something bad" in an individual's psyche, then attempts to describe how an analyst can find it and fix it. Traditional psychoanalytic terms, such as "dysfunction of the ego," "bad object representation," or "low self-esteem," are descriptions of one or another *bad thing* in a patient's mind. Kohut, however, recognized in his clinical work that his patients were more afraid of experiencing *nothing* than they were of suffering the effects of something bad. A world in which a patient has *something* bad—be it memory, fantasy, object relationship, sense of self, or experience—is still better than a world with *nothing*, because the patient has something she can rely on to organize her experience. The world with *nothing* provides the patient with no framework in which to find herself.

In her traumatic environment, Shoko tried to verbalize how her husband was bad. She was extreme in her expression. Like a new-born baby who has not seen what human life is like, Shoko struggled to find a way to describe the kind of world she lived in. We may understand her outsized expression as her effort to outline this new world, and through this expression, she came to experience clearly who she was, how she lived, and what the world was like.

Because Shoko was traumatized, she suffered from divisions between perpetrator and victim, men and women, certain and uncertain. I tried to understand her aggressive attacks against male figures, including me, as her work of mourning her own loss, but this effort failed. My professional attitude became one more subject for her to attack.

In this context of mutual misunderstanding, Shoko's racially-charged speech reminded me of my own traumatic experience abroad. I searched for the right way to react; the best "psychoanalytic way" to treat her. But I was not able to find a certain answer, and I could only access my own painful experience. I wondered if my self-disclosure would be a counter-attack against Shoko, but finally, I revealed it as honestly and gently as I could, and explained why hers were not good words.

This self-disclosure was my surrender to the moment without division between certainty and uncertainty. I thought of the psychoanalytic theories I had learned—some said that I should not self-disclose, some said that I could—but the theories were both right *and* wrong. While I was certain about a particular theory of self-disclosure, I was also *not certain* about the theory. I finally recognized that my focusing on a sense of uncertainty was itself an effort to find a sense of certainty, and vice versa. At the end, I understood that I had avoided putting myself into a vulnerable position.

In our relationship, the vulnerability emerged where our traumatic experiences crossed. Shoko and I were both people who shared the vulnerability of living in this world. We were both treated inhumanly by others, and we treated others inhumanly as well. We could not control the world, but we both lived in it. Sharing it made Shoko access her own painful feelings and made it possible for her to describe how she had experienced being treated inhumanly by her husband.

What is the difference between this attitude and an "optimal analytic stance" suggested by many contemporary analysts (Orange, Atwood, & Stolorow, 1997; Bacal, 2010; Stolorow, 2013; Hoffman, 1998; Renik, 1995, 1998)? An optimal analytic stance is uniquely determined at a particular moment in a particular relationship. But these thinkers are still seeking a *right way* to treat the patient, although they believe that there may be more than one answer. They accept their own fallibility as professional analysts, but they still assume that an "optimal" way exists. Accepting the psychoanalytic zero, in contrast, requires an analyst to suspend the belief that there *is* an optimal answer. It requires the analyst to recognize unpredictability and unknowability in the analytic process and throughout psychoanalytic theories and techniques, and requires her to be aware that her effort to accept a sense of uncertainty as well as certainty around analytic theory stems from her preoccupation with a sense of certainty. The psychoanalytic zero calls on the analyst to surrender herself to the moment without any distinctions, including right or wrong.

We live in the future, from Kohut's point of view, thirty years after his death. We live in the moment, as Kohut (1975) stated, when Freud has finally died and we have lost idealized figures—not only Freud and his followers but also his opponents. For the last thirty years, we have traversed "the vast unexplored area into which the first explorers could make only a few halting steps" (Kohut, 1975, p.328), deconstructing psychoanalytic theories that we have previously relied upon. What we have finally found was that the theories are both certain and uncertain, trustworthy and untrustworthy for us and our patients. The *real* problems and patients we face are too diverse and too individual to be understood *only* through theory. What we have emphasized in this chapter and throughout this book is the need to surrender ourselves to the origin point of human activities, facing our fallibility and vulnerability. This perspective is, I believe, an effort to get back to the discussion about the essence of psychoanalysis, as described by Kohut (1980):

> (Psychoanalysis is) a science that is defined not by the specific theories formulated by Freud's ordering mind … but by the good fortune—the genius of the moment, one might say—of Breuer's and Anna O.'s seminal encounter. It is the basic psychoanalytic situation, in other words, the situation of someone reporting his inner life while, another empathically listens to the report in order to be able to explain it, that defines analysis and not the particular theory or ordering principle that the listener employs.
>
> *(Kohut, 1980, pp.515–516)*

This statement still poses the greatest challenge to us: how can we allow ourselves to be open to any voice from any patient at any moment in any relationship, while we free ourselves from preoccupation, even the preoccupation with being open?

EPILOGUE

This book reflects my thirteen-year struggle, since returning to my country in 2006, to integrate my psychoanalytic training in New York (in English, my second language) with my own practice in Japan. When I was once again able to communicate with my colleagues and patients in Japanese, I immediately felt compelled to address and translate self psychological, intersubjective, and relational concepts and explain them in the context of my native culture. Somewhat to my surprise, I found this was not, and is not, always difficult. For instance, Doi (1962, 1973, 1989) discusses a well-known cultural concept, *amae*—a concept similar to self-selfobject relatedness in Kohutian terms. Self psychology, intersubjective theories, and relational psychoanalysis are recognized in Japanese psychoanalytic circles, but they have not occupied the center of attention as they have in America. It is my impression that in America, most theorists in self psychology, intersubjective theories, and relational psychoanalysis are known to be quite open to cultural diversity, yet the discussion of non-North American cultures is rare in even these psychoanalytic circles. A unique psychological attitude in one culture is de-emphasized in another, and vice versa. The North American and Japanese psychoanalytic circles have been dissociated from each other. I hoped that the process of exploring Japanese terms from self psychological, intersubjective, and relational points of view might be a means to draw them closer together.

Mono no aware is one of the Japanese cultural ideals to which I have paid close attention, because I believe it includes a dynamic systems view. Norinaga Motoori, a linguistic scholar in 18th-century Japan, and other philosophers, consider it to be the essential element in Japanese aesthetics. The phrase is variously translated as "an empathy for things/life/love," "the ah-ness of things/life/love," or "the pathos of things/life/love." A single image is often used to illustrate the concept: *Mono no aware* is what happens when a person experiences the fluttering fall of cherry blossom petals as a movement of the mind. The aesthetics of the term are manifest in any post-medieval Japanese art form, such as *waka* (a twenty-one-syllable Japanese poem), or a Noh play.

For me, however, these translations fall short. They understand the term in an intrapsychic and one-way fashion, and mainly focus on a person experiencing herself as influenced by Nature. But *mono no aware* goes deeper; it includes a person's recognition of herself as a component of a bigger system—Nature, or the cosmic tide of time—where one is influencing and being influenced by the many other components within it. The movement of mind associated with falling petals is a manifestation of "a dance of mutual influence." "For the Japanese, nature is neither to be recognized or analyzed as an object; nor to be artificially reconstructed after being reduced to its elements" (Isobe, 1976, p.102, my translation). A person who knows that in *waka* she "should not describe nature but describe herself in order to create a poem about nature," would be called a person who knows *mono no aware* (Isobe, 1976, p. 107). Through a perturbation in the mind, she can enjoy discovering a sign of transformation in what had, until then, seemed an unchanging nature. In this aesthetic, all components of nature, including oneself, are loosely but optimally coordinated, with each influencing and being influenced. Thus, a human being is never seen as static or discrete.

In the treatment of an obsessive-compulsive Japanese male patient who was intolerant of anyone's mistakes, including his own, we both experienced a strong sense of anxiety. At all times, I was concerned that even my slightest misstep might disappoint him. One day, I tried to cross my legs—probably a self-regulatory effort in this highly tense situation—and failed, and my leg bumped a stool. I said nothing about this clumsiness, but my face expressed the thought, "Oops, I have made a mess of it!" To my surprise, the tension in his body relaxed and he smiled. He said, "I was making you feel nervous, and your mishap changed the chemistry between us." This patient, who sensed a transformation in what had been a too tightly coordinated interaction, could be called a person who knows *mono no aware*.

Psychoanalytic concepts were originally expressed in German within the context of European and Jewish culture. They were carried to the United States and other countries, and have gone on to influence and be influenced by other cultures. Today, this cross-cultural process continues, with new ideas joining and deepening the flow. I can sense *mono no aware* in the writing of this book; I am strongly influenced by this tide of developments, even as I exert my own slight influence on it. The transformation is in process …

REFERENCES

Abe, M. & Heine, S. (1992). *A Study of Dogen: His Philosophy and Religion*. Albany, NY: State University of New York Press.

Adelman, A. (1995). Traumatic memory and the intergenerational transmission of Holocaust narratives. *The Psychoanalytic Study of the Child*, 50(1), 343–367.

Ai, A. L. (2006). Daoist spirituality and philosophy: Implications for holistic health, aging, and longevity. In E. R. Mackenzie (ed.). *Complementary and Alternative Medicine for Older Adults: A Guide to Holistic Approaches to Healthy Aging* (pp.149–160). New York: Springer Publishing Company.

Allport, G. W. (1961). *Pattern and Growth in Personality*. New York: Holt, Rinehart, & Winston.

Amer, A. B. (2013). Informed consent in adult psychiatry. *Oman Medical Journal*, 28(4), 228–231.

Archard, D. (2008). Informed consent: Autonomy and self-ownership. *Journal of Applied Philosophy*, 25(1), 19–34.

Arlow, J. A. (1961). Silence and the theory of technique. *Journal of the American Psychoanalytic Association*, 9, 44–55.

Aron, L. (1996). *A Meeting of Minds*, 2nd ed.Hillsdale, NJ: The Analytic Press.

Aron, L. (1999). Clinical choices and the relational matrix. *Psychoanalytic Dialogue*, 9, 1–29.

Aron, L. (2005). The tree of knowledge: Good and evil conflicting interpretations. *Psychoanalytic Dialogues*, 15(5), 681–707.

Atwood, G. E. (2011). A discussion of philosophy and psychotherapy: Part 3 – epistemology: The darkness of unknowing. *International Journal of Psychoanalytic Self Psychology*, 6(3), 395–404.

Atwood, G. E. & Stolorow, R. D. (1979). *Faces in a Cloud: Intersubjectivity in Personality Theory*. Northvale, NJ: Jason Aronson.

Bacal, H. A. (2006). Specificity theory: Conceptualizing a personal and professional quest for therapeutic possibility. *International Journal of Psychoanalytic Self Psychology*, 1(2), 133–155.

Bacal, H. A. (2010). *The Power of Specificity in Psychotherapy: When Therapy Works and When It Doesn't*. New York: Jason Aronson.

Baraitser, L. (2008). Mum's the word: Intersubjectivity, alterity, and the maternal subject. *Studies in Gender and Sexuality*, 9, 86–110.

Beauchamp, T. L. & Childress, J. F. (1994). *Principles of Biomedical Ethics*, 4th ed.Oxford: Oxford University Press.

Beauchamp, T. L. & Childress, J. F. (2001). *Principles of Biomedical Ethics,* 5th ed. New York: Oxford University Press.

Benjamin, J. (1990). An outline of intersubjectivity: The development of recognition. *Psychoanalytic Psychology*, 7, 33–46.

Benjamin, J. (1995). *Like Subjects, Love Objects: Essays on Recognition and Sexual Difference.* New Haven, CT: Yale University Press.

Benjamin, J. (2004). Beyond doer and done to: An intersubjective view of thirdness. *Psychoanalytic Quarterly*, 73, 5–46.

Benjamin, J. (2007). Intersubjectivity, thirdness, and mutual recognition. Paper presented at the Institute for Contemporary Psychoanalysis, Los Angeles, CA.

Benjamin, J. (2010). Can we recognize each other? Response to Donna Orange. *International Journal of Psychoanalytic Self Psychology*, 5(3), 244–256.

Benjamin, J. (2018). *Beyond Doer and Done To: Recognition Theory, Intersubjectivity and the Third.* New York: Routledge.

Binswanger, L. (1963). *Being-in-the-world: The Selected Papers of Ludwig Binswanger.* J. Needleman (ed.). New York: Basic Books.

Bion, W. (1970). *Attention and Interpretation.* London: Tavistock Publication.

Boris, H. N. (1986). Bion re-visited. *Contemporary Psychoanalysis*, 22(2), 159–184.

Boris, H. N. (1987). Tolerating nothing. *Contemporary psychoanalysis*, 23(3), 351–366.

Boss, M. (1963). *Psychoanalysis and Daseinanalysis.* L. B. Lefebre (trans.). New York: Basic Books.

Boston Change Process Study Group (2007). The foundational level of psychodynamic meaning: Implicit process in relation to conflict, defense and the dynamic unconscious. *International Journal of Psychoanalysis*, 88, 843–860.

Brandchaft, B. (2001). Obsessional disorders: A developmental systems perspective. *Psychoanalytic Inquiry*, 21, 253–288.

Brandchaft, B. (2010). Reflections on the unconscious. In B. Brandchaft, S. Doctors, & D. Sorter (eds.). *Toward an Emancipatory Psychoanalysis: Brandchaft's Intersubjective Vision.* (pp. 221–242). New York: Routledge.

Brandchaft, B., Doctors, S., & Sorter, D. (2010). *Toward an Emancipatory Psychoanalysis: Brandchaft's Intersubjective Vision.* New York: Routledge

Breuer, J. & Freud, S. (1893). On the psychical mechanism of hysterical phenomena: Preliminary communication from studies on hysteria. *The Standard Edition of the Complete Psychological Works of Sigmund Freud* (Vol. 2, pp.1–17), London: Hogarth Press.

Bromberg, P. M. (2009). Truth, human relatedness, and the analytic process: An interpersonal/relational perspective. *The International Journal of Psychoanalysis*, 90(2), 347–361.

Brothers, D. (2008). *Toward a Psychology of Uncertainty: Trauma-Centered Psychoanalysis.* New York: Routledge.

Brothers, D. (2014). War, peace, and promise-making: Becoming a late-life activist. *Psychoanalytic Inquiry*, 34, 766–775.

Brothers, D. & Togashi, K. (2019) After the world collapsed: Two culturally embedded forms of service to others following wide-scale societal traumas. In D. M. Goodman, E. R. Severson, & H. Macdonald (eds.). *Race, Rage, and Resistance: Philosophy, Psychology, and the Perils of Individualism* (pp.198–211). New York: Routledge.

Bugental, J. (1965). *The Search for Authenticity: An Existential-Analytic Approach to Psychotherapy.* New York: Holt, Rinehart & Winston.

Bugental, J. (1967). *Challenges of Humanistic Psychology*. New York: McGraw-Hill.

Carr, R. (2014). Authentic solicitude: What the madness of combat can teach us about authentically being-with our patients. *International Journal of Psychoanalytic Self Psychology*, 9, 115–130.

Caruth, C. (1996). *Unclaimed Experience: Trauma, Narrative, and History*. Baltimore, MD: John Hopkins University Press.

Corpt, E. A. (2013). Peasant in the analyst's chair: Reflections, personal and otherwise, on class and the forming of an analytic identity. *International Journal of Psychoanalytic Self Psychology*, 8, 52–69.

Corpt, E. A. (2016). The complication of caring and ethical turn in psychoanalysis. In. D. M. Goodman & E. R. Severson (eds.). *The Ethical Turn: Otherness and Subjectivity in Contemporary Psychoanalysis* (pp.101–116). New York: Routledge.

Cushman, P. (1995). *Constructing the Self, Constructing America: A Cultural History of Psychotherapy*. Reading, MA: Addison-Wesley.

Cushman, P. (2011). So who's asking? Politics, hermeneutics and individuality. In R. Frie & W. J. Coburn (eds.), *Persons in Context: The Challenge of Individuality in Theory and Practice* (pp.21–40). New York: Routledge.

Deutscher Bundestag (2004). *Zwischenbericht der Enquete-Kommission Ethik und Recht der modernen*. Medizin: Patientenverfügungen.

Disaster Prevention Headquarter of Fukushima Prefecture (2019). Damage situation associated with 2011 Tohoku district-off the Pacific Ocean Earthquake, No.1759, November 5, 2019. Fukushima: Disaster Prevention Division, Fukushima.

Doi, T. (1962). Amae: A key concept for understanding Japanese personality structure. In R. J. Smith & R. K. Beardsley (eds.). *Japanese Culture: Its Development and Characteristics* (pp.132–139). Chicago: Aldine Publishing.

Doi, T. (1973). *The Anatomy of Dependence*, Rev. ed. Tokyo: Kodansha International.

Doi, T. (1989). The concept of amae and its psychoanalytic implication. *International Review of Psycho-Analysis*, 16, 349–354.

Emergency Disaster Countermeasures Headquarters of the National Police Agency (2019). Police countermeasures and damage situation associated with 2011 Tohoku district-off the Pacific Ocean Earthquake, September 10, 2019. Tokyo: National Police Agency.

Ferenczi, S. (1949). Confusion of the tongues between the adults and the child. *International Journal of Psychoanalysis*, 30, 225–230.

Fosshage, J. L. (1995). An expansion of motivational theory: Lichtenberg's motivational systems model. *Psychoanalytic Inquiry*, 15, 421–436.

Frank, A. (1995). *The Wounded Storyteller: Body, Illness and Ethics*. Chicago, IL: University of Chicago Press.

Frankl, V. E. (1946). *Man's Search for Meaning*. Boston, MA: Beacon Press.

Freeman, M. (2002). Charting the narrative unconscious: Cultural memory and the challenge of autobiography. *Narrative Inquiry*, 12, 193–211.

Freeman, M. P. (2012). The narrative unconscious. *Contemporary Psychoanalysis*, 48, 344–366.

Freud, S. (1896). Further remarks on the neuro-psychoses of defence. In *The Standard Edition of the Complete Psychological Works of Sigmund Freud* (Vol. 3, pp.159–188). London: Hogarth Press.

Freud, S. (1898). Sexuality in the aetiology of the neuroses. In *The Standard Edition of the Complete Psychological Works of Sigmund Freud* (Vol. 3, pp.259–285). London: Hogarth Press.

Freud, S. (1900–1901). The interpretation of dreams. In *The Standard Edition of the Complete Psychological Works of Sigmund Freud* (Vol. 4–5). London: Hogarth Press.

Freud, S. (1905a). Three essays on the theory of sexuality. *The Standard Edition of the Complete Psychological Works of Sigmund Freud* (Vol. 7, pp. 125–245). London: Hogarth Press.

Freud, S. (1905b). On psychotherapy. In *The Standard Edition of the Complete Psychological Works of Sigmund Freud* (Vol. 7, pp.255–268). London: Hogarth Press.

Freud, S. (1906). My views on the part played by sexuality in the aetiology of the neuroses. In *The Standard Edition of the Complete Psychological Works of Sigmund Freud* (Vol.7, pp.271–279). London: Hogarth Press.

Freud, S. (1913). Totem and taboo. In *The Standard Edition of the Complete Psychological Works of Sigmund Freud* (Vol. 13, pp.1–161). London: Hogarth Press.

Freud, S. (1914). On the history of the psycho-analytic movement. *The Standard Edition of the Complete Psychological Works of Sigmund Freud* (Vol. 14, pp.1–66). London: Hogarth Press.

Freud, S. (1920a). Beyond the pleasure principle. In *The Standard Edition of the Complete Psychological Works of Sigmund Freud* (Vol. 18, pp.1–64). London: Hogarth Press.

Freud, S. (1920b). A note on the prehistory of the technique of analysis. In *The Standard Edition of the Complete Psychological Works of Sigmund Freud* (Vol. 18, pp.261–265). London: Hogarth Press.

Freud, S. (1923a). Two encyclopaedia articles. In *The Standard Edition of the Complete Psychological Works of Sigmund Freud* (Vol. 18, pp.233–260). London: Hogarth Press.

Freud, S. (1923b). The ego and the id. *The Standard Edition of the Complete Psychological Works of Sigmund Freud* (Vol. 19, pp.12–59). London: Hogarth Press.

Freud, S. (1924). The economic problem of masochism. *The Standard Edition of the Complete Psychological Works of Sigmund Freud* (Vol. 19, pp.155–170). London: Hogarth Press.

Freud, S. (1925a). Some additional notes on dream-interpretation as a whole. *The Standard Edition of the Complete Psychological Works of Sigmund Freud* (Vol. 19, pp.123–138). London: Hogarth Press.

Freud, S. (1925b). An autobiographical study. *The Standard Edition of the Complete Psychological Works of Sigmund Freud* (Vol. 20, pp.3–74). London: Hogarth Press.

Freud, S. (1927). The future of an illusion. *The Standard Edition of the Complete Psychological Works of Sigmund Freud* (Vol. 21, pp.1–56). London: Hogarth Press.

Freud, S. (1930). Civilization and its discontents. *The Standard Edition of the Complete Psychological Works of Sigmund Freud* (Vol. 21, pp.59–145). London: Hogarth Press.

Frie, R. (1997). *Subjectivity and Intersubjectivity in Modern Philosophy and Psychoanalysis: A Study of Sartre, Binswanger, Lacan, and Habermas.* Lanham, MD: Rowman and Littlefield

Frie, R. (2011). Irreducible cultural contexts: German–Jewish experience, identity, and trauma in a bilingual analysis. *International Journal of Psychoanalytic Self Psychology*, 6(2), 136–158.

Frie, R. (2012a). On culture, history, and memory: Encountering the "narrative unconscious". *Contemporary Psychoanalysis*, 48(3), 329–343.

Frie, R. (2012b). Psychoanalysis, religion, philosophy and the possibility of dialogue: Freud, Binswanger and Pfister. *International Forum of Psychoanalysis*, 21, 106–116.

Frie, R. (2016). Psychoanalysis, narrative, and hermeneutics: An integrative account. *Story Worlds*, 8(1), 119–136.

Frie, R. (2017a). *Not in My Family: German Memory and Responsibility After the Holocaust.* New York: Oxford University Press.

Frie, R. (2017b). Understanding history's impact: Or, how to avoid reading the present onto the past. *Psychoanalysis, Self and Context*, 12(3), 269–276.

Frie, R. & Reis, B. (2001). Understanding intersubjectivity: Psychoanalytic formulations and their philosophical underpinnings. *Contemporary Psychoanalysis*, 37(2), 297–327.

Friedman, L. (1982). The humanistic trend in recent psychoanalytic theory. *Psychoanalytic Quarterly*, 51, 353–371.

Fromm, E. (1959). *Sigmund Freud's Mission: An Analysis of His Personality and Influence*. New York: Harper & Brothers.

Fromm, E. (1979). *Greatness and Limitations of Freud's Thought*. New York: Harper & Row.

Fromm, E. (1989). *The Art of Being*. New York: Continuum International Publishing Group.

Fromm, E. (1994). *On Being Human*. New York: Continuum International Publishing Group.

Ghent, E. (1990). Masochism, submission, surrender: Masochism as a perversion of surrender. *Contemporary Psychoanalysis*, 26, 108–136.

Gill, M. M. (1983). The point of view of psychoanalysis: Energy discharge or person? *Psychoanalysis & Contemporary Thought*, 6(4), 523–551.

Gill, M. M. (2000). *Psychoanalysis in Tradition: A Personal View*. Hillsdale, NJ: The Analytic Press.

The Great Hanshin-Awaji Earthquake Memorial Disaster Reduction and Human Renovation Institution (2016). *Disaster Reduction and Human Renovation Institution Pictorial Record 1995.1.17*. Kobe: The Great Hanshin-Awaji Earthquake Memorial Disaster Reduction and Human Renovation Institution .

Greenson, R. R. (1967). *The Technique and Practice of Psychoanalysis, Vol. 1*. New York: International University Press.

Grotstein, J. S. (1999). Melanie Klein and Heinz Kohut: An odd couple or secretly connected? *Progress in Self Psychology*, 15, 123–146.

Guntrip, H. (1971). *Psychoanalytic Theory, Therapy, and the Self*. New York: Basic Books.

Gutkin, D. C. (1973). An analysis of the concept of moral intentionality. *Human Development*, 16(5), 371–381.

Harris, A. (2011). The relational tradition: Landscape and canon. *Journal of the American Psychoanalytic Association*, 59, 701–735.

Herman, J. (1992). *Trauma and Recovery: The Aftermath of Violence – from Domestic Abuse to Political Terror*. New York: Basic Books.

Hermansson, A. R. & Ternestedt, B. M. (2000). What do we know about the dying patient –awareness as a means to improve palliative care. *Medicine and Law*, 19, 335–344.

Hernández-Wolfe, P. (2011). Decolonization and "mental" health: A Mestiza's journey in the borderlands. *Women & Therapy*, 34(3), 293–306.

Hoffman, I. Z. (1998). *Ritual and Spontaneity in the Psychoanalytic Process: A Dialectical-Constructivist View*. Hillsdale, NJ: The Analytic Press.

Hofmann, S. G., Asnaani, A., & Hinton, D. E. (2010). Cultural aspects in social anxiety and social anxiety disorder. *Depression and Anxiety*, 27(12), 1117–1127.

Horney, K. (1950). *Neurosis and Human Growth: The Struggle Toward Self-Realization*. New York: W.W. Norton.

Huppertz, B. (2018). *Approaches to Psychic Trauma: Theory and Practice*. Lanham, MD: Rowman & Littlefield Publishers.

Ishikawa, K. (1938). Sekimon shingagushi ni kansuru Kenkyu. In *Kinshei Nihon Shaki Kyoikushi no Kenkyu* [in Japanese] (pp. 372–550). Tokyo: Toyo Tosho.

Isobe, T. (1976). *Mujo No Kozo* [in Japanese]. Tokyo: Kodansha.

Jacobs, L. (2017). On dignity, a sense of dignity and inspirational shame. *Psychoanalytic Inquiry*, 37(6), 380–394.

Jaenicke, C. (2008). *The Risk of Relatedness: Intersubjectivity Theory in Clinical Practice*. New York: Jason Aronson.

Janoff-Bulman, R. (1992). *Shattered Assumptions: Towards a New Psychology of Trauma*. New York: Free Press.

Jung, C. G. (1921). Psychological types. In *Collected Works of C. G. Jung* (Vol. 6). Princeton, NJ: Princeton University Press, 1971.

Jung, C.G. (1951). Aion: Researches into the phenomenology of the self. In *Collected Works of C. G. Jung* (Vol. 9, Part 2). Princeton, NJ: Princeton University Press, 1969.

Kauffman, J. (2002). Safety and assumptive world: A theory of traumatic loss. In J. Kauffman (ed.). *Loss of the Assumptive World*. New York: Brunner-Routledge.

Kernberg, O. F. (1975). *Borderline Conditions and Pathological Narcissism*. New York: Jason Aronson.

Klein, G. (1976). *Psychoanalytic Theory: An Exploration of Essentials*. Madison, CT: International Universities Press.

Knoblauch, S. H. (2018). Attention and narration to micro-moment registrations of embodied dialogue in the clinical interaction: How are we doing? *Psychoanalytic Inquiry*, 38(7), 502–510.

Kohut, H. (1959), Introspection, empathy and psychoanalysis. In P. H. Ornstein (ed.). *The Search for the Self* (Vol. 1, pp.205–232). New York: International Universities Press.

Kohut, H. (1968). The psychoanalytic treatment of narcissistic personality disorders: Outline of a systematic approach. In P.H. Ornstein (ed.). *The Search for the Self*, (Vol. 1, pp. 477–509). New York: International Universities Press.

Kohut, H. (1971). *The Analysis of the Self*. Madison, CT: International Universities Press.

Kohut, H. (1975). The future of psychoanalysis. *Annual of Psychoanalysis*, 3, 325–340.

Kohut, H. (1977). *The Restoration of the Self*. New York: International Universities Press.

Kohut, H. (1980). Selected problems in self psychology theory. In P. H. Ornstein (ed.). *The Search for the Self* (Vol. 4, pp. 498–523). Madison, CT: International Universities Press.

Kohut, H. (1981). Conversations with Heinz Kohut. In H. Kohut (ed.). *Self Psychology and the Humanities: Reflections on New Psychoanalytic Approach* (pp.215–270). New York: W. W. Norton.

Kohut, H. (1982). Introspection, empathy, and mental health. *International Journal of Psychoanalysis*, 63, 395–408.

Kohut, H. (1984). *How Does Analysis Cure?*Chicago, IL: University of Chicago Press.

Kohut, H. (1985). *Self Psychology and the Humanities: Reflections on New Psychoanalytic Approach*. New York: W. W. Norton.

Kuki, S. (1932). Contingency (Doctoral Dissertation). In *The Complete Works of Kuki Shuzo* (Vol. 2, pp.267–322) [in Japanese]. Tokyo: Iwanami Shoten.

Kuki, S. (1935). The problems of contingency. In *The Complete Works of Kuki Shuzo* (Vol. 2, pp.1–264) [in Japanese]. Tokyo: Iwanami Shoten.

Kuki, S. (1936). Modalities of contingency. In *Philosophy of Contingency and Astonishment* (pp.25–45) [in Japanese]. Tokyo: Shoritsu-Shinsui.

Lannamann, J. W., Harris, L. M., Bakos, A. D., & Baker, K. J. (2008). Ending the end-of-life communication impasse: A dialogic intervention. *Cancer Communication and Aging*, 293–317.

Lee, R. R. & Martin, J. C. (1991). *Psychotherapy after Kohut: A Textbook of Self Psychology*. Hillsdale, NJ: The Analytic Press.

Levenson, E. A. (1974). Changing concepts of intimacy in psychoanalytic practice. *Contemporary Psychoanalysis*, 10(3), 359–369.

Levenson, E. A. (1996). Aspects of self-revelation and self-disclosure. *Contemporary Psychoanalysis*, 32(2), 237–248.

Lichtenberg, J. D. (1985). Humanism and the science of psychoanalysis. *Psychoanalytic Inquiry*, 5(3), 343–367.

Lichtenberg, J. D. (1988). A theory of motivational-functional systems as psychic structures. Journal of the American Psychoanalytic Association, 36S, 57–72.

Lichtenberg, J. D. (1989). *Psychoanalysis and Motivation.* Hillsdale, NJ: The Analytic Press.

Lichtenberg, J. D. (2001). Motivational systems and model scenes with special references to bodily experience. *Psychoanalytic Inquiry*, 21, 430–447.

Lichtenberg, J. D. (2009). Reflections on a contemporary psychoanalytic metatheory. *International Journal of Psychoanalytic Self Psychology*, 4(4), 414–431.

Lichtenberg, J. D. & Kindler, A. R. (1994). A motivational systems approach to the clinical experience. *Journal of American Psychoanalytic Association*, 42, 405–420.

Lichtenberg, J. D., Lachmann, F. M., & Fosshage, J. L. (1992). *Self and Motivational Systems: Towards a Theory of Psychoanalytic Technique*. Hillsdale, NJ: The Analytic Press.

Lichtenberg, J. D., Lachmann, F. M., & Fosshage, J. L. (1996). *The Clinical Exchange*. Hillsdale, NJ: The Analytic Press.

Lichtenberg, J. D., Lachmann, F. M., & Fosshage, J. L. (2011). *Psychoanalysis and Motivational Systems: A New Look*. New York: Routledge.

Loewald, H. (1979). The waning of the Oedipus complex. *Journal of the American Psychoanalytic Association*, 27(4), 751–775.

Lopez, D. S. (1998). *Elaborations of Emptiness: Uses of the Heart Sutra.* Princeton, NJ: Princeton University Press.

Meissner, W. W. (1985). Psychoanalysis: The dilemma of science and humanism. *Psychoanalytic Inquiry*, 5(3), 471–498.

Meissner, W. W. (2003). *Ethical Dimension of Psychoanalysis: A Dialogue*. New York: The State University of New York Press.

Meltzer, D. (1971). Sincerity: A study in the atmosphere of human relations. In *Sincerity and other Works: The Collected Papers of Donald Meltzer* (pp.185–284). London: Karnac Books, 1994.

Mendoza, S. (2010). The O of emptiness and the emptiness of O. *British Journal of Psychotherapy*, 26(3), 305–320.

Miletic, M. J. (1998). Rethinking self-disclosure: An example of the clinical utility of the analyst's self-disclosing activities. *Psychoanalytic Inquiry*, 18(4), 580–600.

Mitchell, S. A. (1988). *Relational Concepts in Psychoanalysis: An Integration*. Cambridge, MA: Harvard University Press.

Mitchell, S. A. (1993). *Hope and Dread in Psychoanalysis*. New York: Basic Books.

Mitchell, S. A. (1997). *Influence and Autonomy in Psychoanalysis*. Hillsdale, NJ: The Analytic Press.

Mitchell, S. A. (2000). *Relationality*. Hillsdale, NJ: The Analytic Press.

Møllgaard, E. (2007). *An Introduction to Daoist Thought: Action, Language, and Ethics in Zhuangzi*. New York: Routledge. Monk, R. (1990). *Ludwig Wittgenstein: The Duty of Genius*. New York: Free Press.

Moore, N. (1983). The archetype of the way: Part 2 the ego-self relationship. *The Journal of Analytical Psychology*, 28(3), 227–252.

Morita, K. (2012). *Sekimon Shingaku to Kindai* [in Japanese]. Tokyo: Yachiyo Shuppan.

Morita, S. (1921). *Shinkeishitsu no Hontai to Ryoho* [in Japanese]. Tokyo: Hakuytsha, 1982.

Murray, M. (2003) Narrative psychology. In J. A. Smith (ed.). *Qualitative Psychology: A Practical Guide to Methods* (pp.111–131). London: SAGE. Nakane, C. & Oishi, S. (1990). *Tokugawa Japan: The Social and Economic Antecedents of Modern Japan* . Tokyo: University of Tokyo Press.

Nishida, K. (1958). *Intelligibility and the Philosophy of Nothingness Three Philosophical Essays*. Honolulu, HI: East-West Center Press, 1966.

Nuland, S. B. (1994). *How We Die: Reflection on Life's Final Chapter.* New York: Knopf.

Obama, Y. (2006). *Kuki Shuzo no Tetsugagu* [in Japanese]. Kyoto: Showado.

Okano, K. (1994). Shame and social phobia: A transcultural viewpoint. *Bulletin of the Menninger Clinic*, 58(3), 323.

Okano, K. (1998). *Haji to Jikoai no Seishin-Bunseki* [in Japanese]. Tokyo: Iwasaki Gakujutsu Shuppansha.

Orange, D. M. (1995). *Emotional Understanding: Studies in Psychoanalytic Epistemology*. New York: The Guilford Press.

Orange, D. M. (2008). Recognition as: Intersubjective vulnerability in the psychoanalytic dialogue. *International Journal of Psychoanalytic Self Psychology*, 3(2), 178–194.

Orange, D. M. (2011). *The Suffering Stranger: Hermeneutics for Everyday Clinical Practice*. New York: Routledge.

Orange, D. M. (2013). Unsuspected shame: Responding to Corpt's "Peasant in the analyst's chair: Reflections, personal and otherwise, on class and the forming of an analytic identity." *International Journal of Psychoanalytic Self Psychology*, 8, 70–76.

Orange, D. M. (2014a). What kind of ethics?: Loewald on responsibility and atonement. *Psychoanalytic Psychology*, 31, 560–569.

Orange, D. M. (2014b). "A psychotherapy for the people: Toward a progressive psychoanalysis" by Lewis Aron and Karen Starr: A book review essay. *International Journal of Psychoanalytic Self Psychology*, 9, 54–66.

Orange, D.M. (2015). *Nourishing the Inner Life of Clinicians and Humanitarians: The Ethical Turn in Psychoanalysis*. New York: Routledge.

Orange, D. M. (2017). The waning of ego and agency: Commentary on Togashi's "Being thrown into the world without informed consent." *Psychoanalysis, Self and Context*, 12(1), 35–39.

Orange, D. M. (2018). Trauma, silence, and dissociation. Paper presented at the Japan Psycho-Analytical Association, 64th Conference, Kyoto, November 25.

Orange, D. M., Atwood, G. E., & Stolorow, R. D. (1997). *Working Intersubjectively: Contextualism in Psychoanalytic Practice*. Hillsdale, NJ: The Analytic Press.

Ornstein, A. (2013) Personal communication. Chicago, October.

O'Neill, O. (2002). *Autonomy and Trust in Bioethics*. Cambridge: Cambridge University Press.

Pastrana, T., Jünger, S., Ostgathe, C., Elsner, F., & Radbruch, L. (2008). A matter of definition – key elements identified in a discourse analysis of definitions of palliative care. *Palliative Medicine*, 22(3), 222–232.

Pateman, C. (2002). Self-ownership and property in the person: Democratization and a tale of two concepts. *Journal of Political Philosophy*, 10(1), 20–53.

Pfeifer, M. P., Sidorov, J. E., Smith, A. C., Boero, J. F., Evans, A. T., Settle, M. B., & EOL Study Group (1994). The discussion of end-of-life medical care by primary care patients and physicians. *Journal of General Internal Medicine*, 9(2), 82–88.

President's Commission for the Study of Ethical Problems in Medicine and Biomedical and Behavioral Research (1982). *Making Health Care Decision: A Report on the Ethical and Legal Implication of Informed Consent in the Patient-Practitioner-Relationship*. Vol. 1. Washington, D. C.: Superintendent of Documents, U.S. Government Printing Office.

Preston, L. & Shumsky, E. (2004). Who tore the web?: Thoughts on psychoanalytic authority and response-ability. *Progress in Self Psychology*, 20, 189–206.

Ragan, S. L., Wittenberg, E., & Hall, H. T. (2003). The communication of palliative care for the elderly cancer patient. *Health Communication*, 15(2), 219–226.

Rank, O. (1924). *The Trauma of Birth* (First published in English in 1929). New York: Routledge, 1994.

Reasoner, P. (1990). Sincerity and Japanese values. *Philosophy East and West*, 40(4), 471–488.

Renik, O. (1995). The ideal of the anonymous analyst and the problem of self-disclosure. *Psychoanalytic Quarterly*, 64, 466–495.

Renik, O. (1998). Getting real in analysis. *Psychoanalytic Quarterly*, 67, 566–593.

Renik, O. (1999). Playing one's cards face up in analysis. *Psychoanalytic Quarterly*, 68, 521–539.

Rogers, C. (1961). *On Becoming a Person: A Therapist's View of Psychotherapy*. London: Constable.

Roland, A. (1996). The influence of culture on the self and selfobject relationships: An Asian-North American comparison. *Psychoanalytic Dialogues*, 6, 461–475.

Ronningstam, E. (2006). Silence: Cultural function and psychological transformation in psychoanalysis and psychoanalytic psychotherapy. *International Journal of Psycho-Analysis*, 87 (5), 1277–1295.

Rorty, R. (1989). *Contingency, Irony, and Solidarity*. Cambridge, UK: Cambridge University Press.

Sagara, T. (1980). *Seijitsu to Nihonjin* [in Japanese]. Tokyo: Pelican Sha.

Sagara, T. (1998a). *Ito Jinsai* [in Japanese]. Tokyo: Pelican Sha.

Sagara, T. (1998b). *Nihonjin no Kokoro to Deau* [in Japanese]. Tokyo: Kadensha.

Sakuma, T. (1977). *Ji-sho-I ron no tenkai: Tojyu kara Banzan* [in Japanese]. *Nihon Shisoshi Kenkyu*, 9, 28–39.

Sarbin, T. R. (1986). *Narrative Psychology: The Storied Nature of Human Conduct*. London: Praeger Press.

Sass, L. A. (1989). Humanism, hermeneutics, and humanistic psychoanalysis: Differing conceptions of subjectivity. *Psychoanalysis and Contemporary Thought*, 12(3), 433–504.

Schafer, R. (1983). *The Analytic Attitude. New edition*. New York: Routledge.

Schafer, R. (1992). *Retelling a Life: Narration and Dialogue in Psychoanalysis*. New York: Basic Books.

Schwartz, W. (1984). The two concepts of action and responsibility in psychoanalysis. *Journal of American Psychoanalytic Association*, 32, 557–572.

Searles, H. F. (1965). *Collected Papers on Schizophrenia and Related Subjects*. Madison, CT: International Universities Press.

Shaw, D. (2014). *Traumatic Narcissism: Relational Systems of Subjugation*. New York: Routledge.

Shengold, L. (1989). *Soul Murder: The Effects of Childhood Abuse and Deprivation*. London: Yale University Press.

Shimokawa, R. (2001). *Kitabatake Chikafusa no Jyugaku* [in Japanese]. Tokyo: Pelican Books.

Spence, D. P. (1982). *Narrative Truth and Historical Truth: Meaning and Interpretation in Psychoanalysis*. London and New York: W.W Norton and Company.

Stern, D. B. (2010). *Partners in Thought: Working with Unformulated Experience, Dissociation, and Enactment*. New York: Routledge.

Stern, D. N. (1992). The "pre-narrative envelope": An alternative view of "unconscious phantasy" in infancy. *Bulletin of the Anna Freud Centre*, 15(4), 291–318.

Stern, S. (2009). The dialectic of empathy and freedom. *International Journal of Psychoanalytic Self Psychology*, 4, 132–164.

Stolorow, R. D. (2007). *Trauma and Human Existence: Autobiographical, Psychoanalytic, and Philosophical Reflections*. New York: Routledge.

Stolorow, R. D. (2008). The contextuality and existentiality of emotional trauma. *Psychoanalytic Dialogues*, 18, 113–123.

Stolorow, R. D. (2010). Ontologizing is not pathologizing: Reply to Ilene Philipson. *International Journal of Psychoanalytic Self Psychology*, 5, 34–36.

Stolorow, R. D. (2011a). *World, Affectivity, Trauma: Heidegger and Post-Cartesian Psychoanalysis*. New York: Routledge.

Stolorow, R. D. (2011b). Individuality in context: the relationality of finitude. In R. Frie & W. Coburn (eds.). *Persons in Context: The Challenge of Individuality in Theory and Practice* (pp. 59–68). New York: Routledge.
Stolorow, R. D. (2012). The renewal of humanism in psychoanalytic therapy. *Psychotherapy*, 49(4), 442–444.
Stolorow, R. D. (2013). Intersubjective-systems theory: A phenomenological-contextualist psychoanalytic perspective. *Psychoanalytic Dialogues*, 23, 383–389.
Stolorow, R. D. & Atwood, G. E. (1992). *Context of Being: The Intersubjective Foundations of Psychological Life*. Hillsdale: NJ: The Analytic Press.
Stolorow, R. D. & Atwood, G. E. (1994). The myth of the isolated mind. *Progress in Self Psychology*, 10, 233–250.
Stolorow, R. D. & Atwood, G. E. (1997). Deconstructing the myth of the neutral analyst: An alternative from intersubjective systems theory. *Psychoanalytic Quarterly*, 66, 431–449.
Stolorow, R. D., Atwood, G. E., & Orange, D. M. (1999). Kohut and contextualism: Toward a post-Cartesian psychoanalytic theory. *Psychoanalytic Psychology*, 16, 380–388.
Stolorow, R. D., Atwood, G. E., & Orange, D. M. (2002). *Worlds of Experience: Interweaving Philosophical and Clinical Dimensions in Psychoanalysis*. New York: Basic Books.
Stolorow, R. D., Brandchaft, B., & Atwood, G. E. (1987). *Psychoanalytic Treatment: An Intersubjective Approach*. Hillsdale, NJ: The Analytic Press.
Stolorow, R. D. & Lachmann, F. M. (1980). *Psychoanalysis of Developmental Arrest: Theory and Treatment*. New York: International Universities Press.
Strozier, C. B. (2001). *Heinz Kohut: The Making of a Psychoanalyst*. New York: Farrar, Straus & Giroux.
Sucharov, M. (2014). Returning to the infinite – Kohut's empathy, Levinas's Other, and the ethical imperative: Discussion of articles by Doris Brothers and Joseph Lichtenberg. *Psychoanalytic Inquiry*, 34, 780–787.
Sullivan, H. S. (1953). *The Interpersonal Theory of Psychiatry*. New York: W. W. Norton.
Suttie, I. D. (1935). *The Origins of Love and Hate*. Middlesex, UK: Peregrine Books, 1963.
Takeuchi, S. (2006). Seijitsu. In K. Oba, T. Inoue, N. Kato, T. Kawakami, S. Kanzaki, T. Shiono, & K. Narita (eds.). *Gendai Rinrigaku Jiten* (pp. 505–506). Tokyo: Kobundo.
Teicholz, J. G. (1998). Self and relationship: Kohut, Loewald, and the postmoderns. *Progress in Self Psychology*, 14, 267–292.
Teicholz, J. G. (2000). The analyst's empathy, subjectivity, and authenticity: Affect as the common denominator. *Progress in Self Psychology*, 16, 33–53.
Terman, M. D. (2013). Personal communication. Chicago, October.
Togashi, K. (2009). A new dimension of twinship selfobject experience and transference. *International Journal of Psychoanalytic Self Psychology*, 4, 21–39.
Togashi, K. (2010). An effort to find self psychological concepts in an Asian culture. *International Journal of Psychoanalytic Self Psychology*, 5(1), 113–115.
Togashi, K. (2012). Mutual finding oneself and not-oneself in the other as a twinship experience. *International Journal of Psychoanalytic Self Psychology*, 7(3), 352–368.
Togashi, K. (2014a). Is it a problem for us to Say, "It is a coincidence that the patient does well"? *International Journal of Psychoanalytic Self Psychology*, 9(2), 87–100.
Togashi, K. (2014b). From search for a reason to search for a meaning: Response to Discussant. *International Journal of Psychoanalytic Self Psychology*, 9(2), 108–114.
Togashi, K. (2014c). A sense of "being human" and twinship experience. *International Journal of Psychoanalytic Self Psychology*, 9(4), 265–281.
Togashi, K. (2014d). Certain and uncertain aspects of a trauma: Response to Doris Brothers. *International Journal of Psychoanalytic Self Psychology*, 9(4), 289–296.

Togashi, K. (2014e). The value of living with uncertainty and its relevance for analytic work: The future of psychoanalysis. Paper presented for the 2014 Taiwan Self Psychology Conference, Taipei, December.

Togashi, K. (2016a). From traumatized individuality to being human with others. Paper presented at the 39th Annual Conference of International Association for Psychoanalytic Self Psychology, Boston, October.

Togashi, K. (2016b). The motivational system of moving toward nothingness. Paper presented at the 2016 Taiwan Self Psychology Conference, Tapei, December.

Togashi, K. (2017a). Being thrown into the world without informed consent. *Psychoanalysis, Self and Context*, 12(1), 20–34.

Togashi, K. (2017b). Creating a space for responsibility: Reply to commentary of Donna Orange. *Psychoanalysis, Self and Context*, 12(1), 40–44.

Togashi, K. (2017c). Beyond the guilt of being: Surrender to the psychoanalytic zero. Paper presented at the 14th Annual IARPP Conference, Sydney, May.

Togashi, K. (2017d). Narrative as the zero: The vacuum state from which the world emerges in a psychoanalytic relationship. Paper presented at the 14th Annual IARPP Conference, Sydney, May.

Togashi, K. (2017e). An Asian ethical perspective on sincerity in psychoanalysis. Paper presented at the Psychology & the Other 2017 Conference, Boston,October.

Togashi, K. (2017f). Therapeutic sincerity in the intersubjective field. Paper presented at the 40th Annual Conference of International Association for Psychoanalytic Self Psychology, Chicago, October.

Togashi, K. (2017g). Surrender to the psychoanalytic zero: The analyst's taking responsibility, telling, and being Makoto. Paper presented at the 2017 Taiwan Self Psychology Conference, Taipei, December.

Togashi, K. (2019a). Surrender and silence: The problem of narrative and non-narrative in psychoanalysis. *Psychoanalysis, Self and Context*, published online.

Togashi, K. (2019b). Trauma, contingency and the psychoanalytic zero. Paper presented at the 42nd IAPSP Annual International Conference, Vancouver, October.

Togashi, K. & Kottler, A. (2012a). The many faces of twinship: From the psychology of the self to the psychology of being human. *International Journal of Psychoanalytic Self Psychology*, 7(3), 331–351.

Togashi, K. & Kottler, A. (2012b). "I am afraid of seeing your face": Trauma and the dread of engaging in a twinship tie. Paper presented at the 10th Anniversary Conference on the International Association for Relational Psychoanalysis and Psychotherapy, New York, March.

Togashi, K. & Kottler, A. (2013). Being human and not being human: The evolution of a twinship experience. Paper presented at the 36th Annual Confernece on the Psychology of the Self, Chicago, October.

Togashi, K. & Kottler, A. (2015). *Kohut's Twinship Across Cultures: The Psychology of Being Human*. London & New York: Routledge.

Togashi, K. & Kottler, A. (2019). Contemporary self psychology and its treatment of traumatized patients. In B. Huppertz (ed.). *Approaches to Psychic Trauma: Theory and Practice* (pp.323–332). Lanham, MD: Rowman & Littlefield Publishers.

Tolstoy, L. (1886). The death of Ivan Ilych. In L. Maude and A. Maude (trans.). *Ivan Ilych, Hadji Murad, and Other Stories*. London: Oxford University Press, 1959.

Turco, R. N. (2014). Traumatic narcissism: Relational systems of subjugation, by Daniel Shaw, Routledge, New York and London, 2013. *Psychodynamic Psychiatry*, 42 (4), 721–725.

Uchinuma, Y. (1977). *Taijinkyfu no Ningengaku* [in Japanese]. Tokyo: Kyobundo.

Uchinuma, Y. (1981). Taijnkyofu no Rinriteki Hensen [in Japanese]. In S. Iida, H. Iwai, & K. Yoshimatsu (eds.). *Taijinkyofu*. Tokyo: Yuhikaku.

Uchinuma, Y. (1983) *Haji no Kozo* [in Japanese]. Tokyo: Kinokuniya Shoten.

Van Der Heide, N. (2007). Authenticity and psychoanalytic technique: A reconsideration. *International Journal of Psychoanalytic Self Psychology*, 2, 275–289.

Walker, A. D. M. (1978). The ideal of sincerity. *Mind*, 87(348), 481–497.

Watsuji, T. (1952). *Nihon Rinri Shisoshi, Vol.2* [in Japanese]. Tokyo: Iwanami.

Weisel-Barth, J. (2015). An ethical vision: Response to Drozek's "The Dignity in Multiplicity." *Psychoanalytic Dialogues*, 25, 463–471.

Winnicott, D. W. (1956). Primary maternal preoccupation. In *Through Paediatrics to Psychoanalysis* (pp.300–305). London: Hogarth Press.

Wittgenstein, L. (1953). *Philosophical Investigations*. G. E. M. Anscombe (trans.). 3rd ed. New York: Macmillan, 1958.

Zahavi, D. (2005). *Subjectivity and Selfhood: Investigating the First-Person Perspective*. Cambridge, MA: MIT Press.

INDEX